INTERMITTENT FASTING FOR WOMEN OVER 50

The Complete Guide for Beginners to Lose Weight, Regain Energy, Delay Aging and Rejuvenate Body with 100 Recipes and a 30-Day Meal Plan

NATHALIE HARTER

© Copyright 2022 by Nathalie Harter - All rights reserved.

The content contained within this book may not be reproduced, duplicated or transmitted without direct written permission from the author or the publisher.

Under no circumstances will any blame or legal responsibility be held against the publisher, or author, for any damages, reparation, or monetary loss due to the information contained within this book. Either directly or indirectly.

Legal Notice:

This book is copyright protected. This book is only for personal use. You cannot amend, distribute, sell, use, quote or paraphrase any part, or the content within this book, without the consent of the author or publisher.

Disclaimer Notice:

Please note the information contained within this document is for educational and entertainment purposes only. All effort has been executed to present accurate, up to date, and reliable, complete information. No warranties of any kind are declared or implied. Readers acknowledge that the author is not engaging in the rendering of legal, financial, medical or professional advice. The content within this book has been derived from various sources. Please consult a licensed professional before attempting any techniques outlined in this book.

By reading this document, the reader agrees that under no circumstances is the author responsible for any losses, direct or indirect, which are incurred as a result of the use of information contained within this document, including, but not limited to, — errors, omissions, or inaccuracies.

Table of Contents

INTRODUCTION 9

CHAPTER 1: BASICS OF INTERMITTENT FASTING 11

    How Does It Work? 12

    The Science Behind Intermittent Fasting 13

CHAPTER 2: METHODS OF INTERMITTENT FASTING 14

    The 16:8 Method 14

    The 14:10 Method 14

    The 5:2 Method 15

    Eat-Stop-Eat Protocol 16

    Alternate Day Fasting 16

    Spontaneous Meal Skipping 17

CHAPTER 3: HEALTH BENEFITS OF INTERMITTENT FASTING 18

    Weight Loss 18

    Tackles Diabetes 18

    Sleep 18

    Resistance to Illnesses 18

    A Healthy Heart 19

    A Healthy Gut 19

    Reduces Inflammation 19

    Promotes Cell Repair 19

    Higher Concentration and Brain Power 19

    Promotes Autophagy and Protects Neurons 20

    Reduced Risk of Depression 20

    Fosters Immune Regulation 21

    Reduces the Risk of Chronic Disease 21

    Improves Genetic Repair Mechanisms 21

    Reduce the Likelihood of Developing Cancer 21

CHAPTER 4: BEST WAY TO DO IT IN MENOPAUSE 23

    What Happens to the Body of a Menopausal Woman? 23

    The Ideal Diet for Menopause 24

CHAPTER 5: FOODS TO CONSUME AND THOSE TO AVOID 25

What to Eat 25

    Berries...25

    Cruciferous Vegetables...25

    Eggs 25

    Fish...25

    Healthy Starches Like Individual Potatoes (With Skins!)..............26

    Legumes 26

    Nuts 26

    Probiotics Help Boost Your Gut Health 26

    Vegetables That Are Rich in Healthy Fats 26

    Water, Water, Water, and More Water 26

What to Avoid 27

    Grains..27

    Starchy Vegetables and Legumes...27

    Sugary Fruits 27

    Milk and Low-Fat Dairy Products 27

    Cashews, Pistachios, and Chestnuts 27

    Most Natural Sweeteners 28

    Alcohol..28

CHAPTER 6: MISTAKES TO AVOID 29

    Going All-in..29

    Binging Before and After Fasting 29

    Fasting Too Often 30

    Not Fasting Enough 30

    Falling Into a Predictable Routine 30

    Pay Attention to Macronutrients...30

    Don't Get Greedy in the Fasting Windows 31

    Don't Try to Rush the Process..31

    Perseverance Is the Key 31

    Don't Frame Unrealistic Expectations 32

CHAPTER 7: TIPS AND TRICKS...33

    Ensure You Are Fasting in a Healthy Way 33

    Obtain Proper Nutrition and Rest 33

    Add Some Exercise...34

    Increase Your Water Intake 34

    Pay Attention to Your Body 34

Avoid Stress 35

Increase Protein Intake 35

Select the Foods You Eat Wisely 35

Consider Supplementation 35

Avoid Overdoing It in the Beginning 36

Find Something to Do When You Fast 36

Detoxify your Body 36

CHAPTER 8: FAQ 37

CHAPTER 9: MEAL PLAN FOR 30 DAYS 40

CHAPTER 10: BREAKFAST 43

1. Avocado Egg Bowls 43

2. Buttery Date Pancakes 43

3. Low Carb Pancake Crepes 44

4. Chia Seed Banana Blueberry Delight 45

5. Egg Omelet 45

6. Savory Breakfast Muffins 46

7. Green Pineapple 47

8. Wholesome Mushroom and Cauliflower Risotto 47

9. Morning Meatloaf 48

10. Keto Oatmeal 48

11. Cinnamon and Pecan Porridge 49

12. Awesome Oatmeal 49

13. Grapefruit Yogurt Parfait 50

14. Creamy Mango and Banana Overnight Oats 50

15. Bacon and Eggs with Tomatoes 51

16. Cinnamon Porridge 52

17. Sesame-Seared Salmon 52

18. Eggs and Salsa 53

19. Poached Egg 53

20. Cheesy Egg Muffins 53

CHAPTER 11: LUNCH 55

21. Salmon with Sauce 55

22. Butter Chicken 55

23. Lamb Curry 56

24. Zuppa Toscana with Cauliflower 57

25. Pork Carnitas 57

26. Cheesy Taco Skillet 58

27. Mini Thai Lamb Salad Bites 58

28. Bacon Egg and Sausage Cups 59

29. Smoked Salmon and Avocado Stacks 59

30. Homemade Turkey Burger and Relish 60

31. Butternut Squash Risotto 61

32. Chicken in Sweet and Sour Sauce with Corn Salad 61

33. Asparagus and Pistachios Vinaigrette 62

34. Chinese Chicken Salad 63

35. Garlic Butter Beef Steak 64

36. Instant Pot Teriyaki Chicken 65

37. Teriyaki Salmon 65

38. Creamy Lamb Korma 66

39. Simple Roasted Cabbage 66

CHAPTER 12: DINNER 68

40. Maple Walnut-Glazed Black-Eyed Peas with Collard Greens 68

41. Filipino Chicken Adobo 69

42. Kale & Artichoke Soup 69

43. Poached Eggs and Bacon on Toast 70

44. Asparagus and Green Peas Salad 70

45. Quick and Easy Squash Soup 71

46. Sesame-Ginger Chicken Salad 71

47. Reds Salad on Bacon and Balsamic Vinaigrette 72

48. Veggie-Stuffed Omelet 73

49. Roasted Carrots and Cashew Salad on Lemon Vinaigrette 73

50. Turmeric Tofu Scramble 74

51. Raspberry Jam and Peanut Butter Overnight Oats 74

52. Roasted Broccoli with Lemon, Garlic and Toasted Pine Nuts 75

53. Vegan Lentil Burger 76

54. Savory Oatmeal Bowl 76

55. Vegan Coconut Kefir Banana Muffins 77

56. Chicken Tetrazzini 78

57. Meatloaf 78

58. Mixed Vegetables and Chicken Egg Rolls 79

59. Chili Cod 80

60. Parsley Tuna Bowls 80

CHAPTER 13: SOUPS 81

61. Creamy Broccoli and Cauliflower Soup 81
62. Chicken Turnip Soup 81
63. Garlicky Chicken Soup 82
64. Cauliflower Curry Soup 82
65. Beef Taco Soup 83
66. Creamy Tomato Soup 84
67. Creamy Broccoli and Leek Soup 84
68. Chicken Soup 85
69. Wild Mushroom Soup 85
70. Roasted Butternut Squash Soup 86
71. Zucchini Cream Soup 86
72. Cauli Soup 87
73. Thai Coconut Soup 87
74. Chicken Ramen Soup 88

CHAPTER 14: DESSERTS 89

75. Baked Apples 89
76. Pumpkin Ice Cream 89
77. Avocado Pudding 90
78. Chocolate Mousse 90
79. Apple Crisp 91
80. Chocolate Crunch Bars 91
81. Homemade Protein Bar 92
82. Shortbread Cookies 92
83. Peanut Butter Bars 93
84. Zucchini Bread Pancakes 93
85. Berry Sorbet 94
86. Quinoa Porridge 94
87. Apple Quinoa 95
88. Kamut Porridge 95
89. Overnight "Oats" 96
90. Blueberry Cupcakes 96
91. Brazil Nut Cheese 97

CHAPTER 15: SNACKS 98

92. Squash Bites 98
93. Pepperoni Bites 98

94. **Party Meatballs** 99

95. **Artichoke Petals Bites** 99

96. **Stuffed Beef Loin in Sticky Sauce** 100

97. **Eggplant Fries** 100

98. **Parmesan Crisps** 101

99. **Roasted Broccoli** 101

100. **Almond Flour Muffins** 102

Conclusion 103

INTRODUCTION

Fasting is an ancient practice that has been practiced by many cultures and religions, such as Islam's month-long Ramadan or the Jewish Yom Kippur. In a nutshell, intermittent fasting means not ingesting any calories for extended periods. While most people think of this as abstaining from all food and liquid, it can also consist of restricting calorie intake on certain days, which is called intermittent fasting.

It has been found to have many benefits for both men and women: improved weight loss; better blood sugar control; increased focus; improved skin complexion; weight maintenance; reduced anxiety, depression and blood pressure.

Intermittent fasting is particularly effective for older adults, as it helps improve insulin sensitivity which promotes a healthy metabolism and helps the body better utilize blood sugar.

Intermittent fasting is also great for hormonal health. By helping optimize insulin sensitivity and blood sugar levels, your hormones can run more efficiently. This includes helpful hormones like leptin that help manage your appetite and ghrelin, which stimulates your body's hunger response. These hormones are critical in managing weight by getting you into a healthy calorie-burning balance.

Women and Intermittent Fasting

There are different types of intermittent fasting, yet it is most effective if done daily. One of the ways that women can do this is to have a fast day and eat according to their body's needs. Does this sound like you?

A fast day means you have one day where you don't eat any food or drink anything but water. You might consider fasting every other day, alternating with non-fast days, where you eat as much as feels good for your body. How long should these fasting days be? It can vary based on how clean your diet has been and how many calories that meal the prior day has. Ideally, it will be from 10 to 14 hours. The general recommendation is not to go over 16 hours.

As you can imagine, older women may find fasting difficult and should consult their health care practitioner before trying any form of fasting. Women who are pregnant or breastfeeding should also consult their physician before trying a fast day.

Remember, this is not an extreme form of fasting. The goal is to simply help you realize how you feel when you are not eating or drinking anything. You may be surprised at the benefits that can come from a 10-12-hour fast day.

This type of intermittent fasting will also show you how much food is truly necessary for sustaining yourself daily. You can then work to incorporate and minimize your food intake while still eating the foods you enjoy.

Keep this in mind, however: the results of fasting do not come from skipping a meal or eating less. They come from changing to a healthier lifestyle that includes healthier foods and portion sizes.

Another great way to get some of the benefits of fasting is to simply restrict your calorie intake on a given day. This can be done by restricting your daily calorie intake by 20 percent. While this is more than what most experts recommend, if you are already eating well and working out regularly, it may be the perfect kick-start to your weight loss journey.

The first fast day in this protocol is generally done one to two weeks after the beginning of your weight loss journey. This way, if you are already on a meal plan, you will soon be able to begin incorporating fasting into your lifestyle. If you are not on a meal plan, I would recommend consulting with your health care professional before starting the intermittent fasting protocol.

CHAPTER 1: BASICS OF INTERMITTENT FASTING

Basically, Fasting is defined as abstaining from eating anything. It is the deliberate action of depriving the body of any form of food for more than six hours.

Whereas Intermittent fasting is a nutritional strategy that provides for a more or less long interval of fasting over a few days, alternating with a period in which you can take food without being too enslaved to the weights but still taking into account some precautions. Intermittent fasting does not need to be carried out every day, but you can choose the different ways suitable for your goals and lifestyles.

In the hours of feeding, it is possible to consume almost all foods giving preference to low-calorie foods such as meat, fish, eggs, limiting simple sugars and choosing those with a low glycemic index, bread pasta, and rice possibly whole grains, legumes, dried and fresh fruits, and good fats.

One of its forms is where the fast is carried out in a cyclic manner to reduce the overall caloric intake in a day.

The main goal is to divert the body's attention from the digestion of food. During the fasting period, in fact, a series of metabolic changes take place in the body: since there is no food left in the stomach to digest, the body focuses on the process of recovery and maintenance.

To most people, it may sound unhealthy and damaging for the body, but scientific research has proven that fasting can produce positive results on the human mind and body. According to Healthline, the American medical-scientific journal, this system helps reduce overall calorie intake and as a result not only can help people lose weight effortlessly but can improve the overall functioning of metabolism. It can also positively affect our mind teaching self-discipline and fighting against bad eating practices and habits. It is basically an umbrella term that is used to define all voluntary forms of fasting. This dietary approach does not restrict the consumption of certain food items; rather, it works by reducing the overall food intake, leaving enough space to meet the essential nutrients the body needs. Therefore, it is proven to be far more effective and much easier in implementation, given that the dieter completely understands the nature and science of intermittent fasting.

Intermittent fasting is categorized into three broad methods of food abstinence, including alternate-day fasting, daily restrictions, and periodic fasting. The means may vary, but the end goal of intermittent fasting remains the same, which is to achieve a better metabolism, healthy body weight, and active lifestyle. The American Heart Association, AHA, has also studied intermittent fasting and its results. According to the AHA, it can help in countering insulin resistance, cardio-metabolic diseases, and leads to weight loss. However, a question mark remains on the sustainability of this health-effective method. The 2019 research "Effects of intermittent fasting on health, aging, and disease" has also found intermittent fasting to be effective against insulin resistance, inflammation, hypertension, obesity, and dyslipidemia. However, the work on this dietary approach is still underway, and the traditional methods of fasting which existed for almost the entire human history, in every religion from Buddhism to Jainism, Orthodox Christianity, Hinduism, and Islam, are studied to found relevance in today's age of science and technology.

How Does It Work?

Eating is a primary need that we satisfy unceasingly from birth. Every day we introduce food into our organism. When we eat, the metabolism activates itself to start the digestive process. This process uses a huge amount of energy. The more food we introduce, the more the body will have to work to metabolize it. If the food is introduced and too much, or too full of sugars and fats the effort that the digestive system must sustain and yet greater.

When we fast, however, we stop this process and this energy dispensing. The saved energy is thus diverted to other metabolic processes, essentially of a restorative type.

Dr. Longo, Director of the Institute of Longevity at the University of Southern California, explained how, thanks to this practice: "the immune system frees itself from useless, unnecessary cells, while it is driven to put back into action naturally, as was the case at the moments of birth and growth, stem cells capable of ensuring regeneration."

The body not engaged in food digestion can better devote itself to its purification by moving toxins away through its emunctory organs. These large internal cleanings obviously have positive repercussions on the state of health of organs and tissues. The organism is detoxified and revitalized.

American researchers at Yale's School of Medicine highlighted how during the break from food, our organism produces a substance capable of extinguishing chronic inflammation. It is called the β-hydroxybutyrate (BHB) and it is capable turn falls into a complex set of proteins that guide the inflammatory response in many pathologies, including several autoimmune diseases. A good result suggests how in the future therapeutic fasting can be used in the early treatment of many inflammatory-based diseases.

Intermittent fasting is a tool that can help us activate the processes described above and face a real fast. In fact, it works between alternating periods of eating and fasting. It is a much more flexible approach, as there are many options to choose from according to body type, size, weight goals, and nutritional needs.

The human body works like a synchronized machine that requires sufficient time for self-healing and repair. When we constantly eat junk and unhealthy food or too high a quantity of food without the consideration of our caloric needs, it leads to obesity and toxic build-up in the body. That is why fasting comes as a natural means of detoxifying the body and providing it enough time to utilize its fat deposits.

Whatever the human body consumes is ultimately broken into glucose, which is later utilized by the cells in glycolysis to release energy. As the blood glucose level rises, insulin is produced to lower the levels and allow the liver to carry out De Novo Lipogenesis, the process in which the excess glucose is turned into glycogen and ultimately stored into fat, resulting in obesity. Intermittent fasting seems to reverse this process by deliberately creating energy deprivation, which is then fulfilled by breaking down the existing fat deposits.

Intermittent fasting works through lipolysis; though it is a natural body process, it can only be initiated when the blood glucose levels drop to a sufficiently low point. That point can be achieved through fasting and exercising. When a person cuts off the external glucose supply for several hours, the body switches to lipolysis. This process of breaking the fats also releases other by-products like ketones which are capable of reducing the oxidative stress of the body and help in its detoxification.

Mark Mattson, a neuroscientist from Johns Hopkins Medicine University, has studied intermittent fasting for almost 25 years of his career. He laid out the workings of intermittent fasting by clarifying its clinical application and the science behind it. According to him, intermittent fasting must be chosen for a healthy lifestyle.

While discussing the application of this dietary approach, it is imperative to understand how intermittent fasting stands out from casual dieting practices. It is not mere abstinence from eating. What is eaten in this dietary lifestyle is equally important as the fasting itself. It does not result in malnutrition; rather, it promotes healthy eating along with the fast. Intermittent fasting is divided into two different states that follow one another. The cycle starts with the "FED" state, which is followed by a "Fasting" state. The duration of the fasting state and the frequency of the FED state are established by the method of intermittent fasting. The latter is characterized by high blood glucose levels, whereas during the fasting state the body goes through a gradual decline in glucose levels. This decline in glucose signals the pancreas and the brain to meet the body's energy needs by processing the available fat molecules. However, if the fasting state is followed by a FED state in which a person binge eats food rich in carbs and fats, it will turn out to be more hazardous for their health. Therefore, the fasting period must be accompanied by a healthy diet.

The Science Behind Intermittent Fasting

Biologically, intermittent fasting works at many levels, from cellular levels to gene expression and body growth. In order to understand the science behind the workings of intermittent fasting, it is important to learn about the role of insulin levels, human growth hormones, cellular repair, and gene expression. Intermittent fasting firstly lowers glucose levels, which in turn drops insulin levels. This lowering of insulin helps fat burning in the body, thus gradually curbing obesity and related disorders. Controlled levels of insulin are also responsible for preventing diabetes and insulin resistance. On the other hand, intermittent fasting boosts the production of human growth hormones up to five times. The increased production of HGH aids quick fat burning and muscle formation.

During the fasting state, the body goes into the process of self-healing at cellular levels, thus removing the unwanted, non-functional cells and debris. This creates a cleansing effect that directly or indirectly nourishes the body and allows it to grow under reduced oxidative stress. Likewise, fasting even affects the gene expression within the human body. The cell functions according to the coding and decoding of the gene's expression; when this transcription occurs at a normal pace in a healthy environment, it automatically translates into the longevity of the cells, and fasting ensures unhindered transcription. Thus, intermittent fasting fights aging, cancer, and boosts the immune system by strengthening the body cells.

CHAPTER 2: METHODS OF INTERMITTENT FASTING

There are several Intermittent Fasting techniques and picking the most appropriate for your case is the first step towards success.

The 16:8 Method

The 16:8 method involves ingesting foods and calorie-containing liquids to an eight-hour window each day and fasting for the remaining 16 hours.

This is probably the most popular fasting method; it is hard to commit mistakes, if not intentionally since the schedule is clear. In addition, the 8-hour eating window can be decided in advance to adapt to your work and personal needs.

This cycle can be repeated as many times as you wish. It is highly suggested to start just once or twice per week to give your body time to adapt to this method. Then, as you gain confidence, you can attempt it for a week or more, depending on your needs.

The first thing to do to get started is pick your eight-hour window. The two most common choices are:

12 am to 8 pm
9 am to 5 pm

If you decide to use the 12 am - 8 pm window, most of the Fasting will happen during the night, and the only real change to your lifestyle will be avoiding evening snacks and skipping breakfast.

Choosing instead the 9 am - 5 pm window, you can have a rich breakfast, lunch, and a light early dinner or a late afternoon snack. However, you can experiment and pick the time frame that best fits your schedule.

16:8 intermittent fasting is probably the more straightforward method to follow and will help you save some money and time on cooking food each week. In addition, this method is not too stressful for the body and can be easily followed.

The biggest drawback of this and other IF methods is overeating. As already said, during the eating window, some people could start to eat more than usual, leading to weight gain and digestive problems.

I suggest beginners start with the 16:8 approach and move into more challenging methods only when your body has fully adapted to this new lifestyle. In most cases, the 16:8 approach will already lead to excellent results.

The 14:10 Method

In some cases, starting with the 16:8 method is too complicated, or your body does not respond as you would expect to the diet. To avoid possible side effects caused by intermittent Fasting and relieve the pressure on your body, it is possible to switch to a 14:10 method.

This method is perfect for people who want to start gradually and is perfectly sustainable even for very long periods as it involves minimal changes to their lifestyle.

Unlike the 16:8 method, the eating window is longer (10 hours). This guarantees greater flexibility in managing meals and the possibility of having three meals a day without stringent time limits.

There are different eating windows that you could try; the most commons are:

> 7 am to 5 pm
> 8 am to 7 pm

There is enough time for a rich breakfast, a balanced lunch, and a light early dinner in both cases.

The 5:2 Method

The 5:2 diet is a calorie-limiting diet that follows a prescriptive program based on days of the week.

This method is particularly effective for very busy people who find it difficult to organize themselves with a fixed eating window during the week. The idea behind the 5:2 method is based on eating five days a week and substantially reducing calories consumed the remaining two days.

5:2 can be considered a part-time diet that does not impose strict restrictions for most of the week, allowing us to eat chocolate, pasta, or any food we desire for five days. Obviously, to avoid nullifying the chances of success of this diet, the recommendation is to consume a normal number of calories during the week and avoid falling into the phenomenon of overeating.

During the two days of calories restrictions, calorie intake should be limited to 500 calories for women and 600 for men. During the other five days, you should aim to consume around 2000 calories per day. This means that you are seeking to consume 3000 calories less or even more in an entire week. Your 500-calorie days will help regulate hunger and insulin levels, naturally reducing your appetite, making it easier to meet the 2000 calorie limit for five days of the week.

There will be no restrictions on the type of food we want to consume; the important thing is not to exceed the number of calories indicated. In terms of weight loss, following this diet strictly, a woman over 50 can expect to lose more or less 5 lb. per week.

This diet method is not particularly intensive for the body, and for this reason, it can also be continued for long periods or until you reach the ideal weight.

If you feel that your goals are too ambitious, you can decide to do two or more cycles to insert some breaks between them so as not to make the diet too stressful. The duration of the breaks can vary; I recommend a week so as not to lose the healthy habits you have built.

Scheduling your meals during a 5:2 diet is not strictly required, but it might help achieve better results. I suggest keeping your meals in 12 hours, between 7 am and 7 pm, avoiding late dinners. A stricter time window can be used if you look for faster results – i.e., from 7 am to 3 pm. By eating earlier in the day and extending the overnight fast, you will significantly help your metabolism.

For your 2000-calories days, you have the freedom to eat whatever you like; I have added to this book 100 healthy recipes that can help you organize your meal plan.

During your 500-calories days, you have to pay more attention to your diet, as it is very easy to reach and exceed 500 calories. Therefore, I suggest you focus on the following foods that usually guarantee a balanced calorie intake and allow you to create delicious recipes:

Vegetables
Fish
Eggs
Small portions of lean meat
Soups

It is recommended to drink only water, but herbal tea and black coffee can be consumed if you want something different.

Eat-Stop-Eat Protocol

This method consists of fasting for 24 hours, twice a week, then eating "responsibly" for the other five days.

Eat-stop-eat falls in the group of methods associated with Intermittent Fasting dieting; unlike regular diets, calorie counting plays a secondary role with this method. Given the time restrictions, it becomes much more difficult to cheat and consume more calories than you should. Obviously, a minimum of willpower is required to respect the fasting periods and not overeat in the periods in which eating is allowed.

With eat stop eat, you can organize your week as you prefer; the important thing is to have two non-consecutive fasting days. This could be confusing at first, but you will always eat something on any calendar day when you adopt this method. For example, if you fast from 8 am on Tuesday to 8 am on Wednesday, you will try to have a meal just before 8 am on Tuesday and eat your next meal just after 8 am on Wednesday, fasting precisely 24 hours.

During fasting days, it is essential to maintain a high level of hydration. Therefore, especially if you decide to "eat stop eating" during hot periods, make an effort to drink frequently.

Like other Intermittent Fasting methods, eating stop eat acts on the metabolism; our body, when it is in a state of fasting for 12-36 hours, will begin to consume the glucose and then move on to burning fat.

Alternate Day Fasting

Like most of the methods of Intermittent Fasting, this technique is straightforward to apply. On this diet, you fast every other day, but there are no restrictions on what you can eat on the non-fasting days.

You are free to drink as much as you want during the fasting days, but you must limit yourself only to water, unsweetened coffee, and unsweetened tea. Any other type of drink should be avoided so as not to compromise the diet. Moreover, during the fasting days, it is allowed to consume about 500 calories.

If this approach sounds similar to the 5:2 method, you are right; you can consider alternate day fasting as a more challenging version of the 5: 2 method.

When and how you decide to consume your calories, the allowance does not affect the results obtained.

This method is more suitable for some people who, due to their multiple commitments, find it challenging to manage strict time constraints in their diet since you can freely decide how and when to consume the calories of the day.

We reduce calories to 500 on fasting days instead of completely zeroing them out to be able to maintain such a diet for more extended periods. Consuming zero calories could bring more significant benefits in terms of weight loss and body purification in the short term but have adverse effects on our body during a prolonged diet.

In terms of weight loss, following this method, you can expect a loss of between 3% and 8% of your body weight over a period of 2 to 12 weeks. The reason for all this variance in results lies in the boundary conditions. For example, an obese and physically active person will tend to lose much more than a slightly overweight person who does not engage in physical activity.

As I said before, you can structure your fasting days as you like in terms of calorie breakdown and what to eat during meals. In my experience, I have seen people handling better fasting days using one of the following approaches:

> One "big" meal in the late afternoon to consume all 500 calories.
> One "big" meal at lunchtime to consume all 500 calories.
> Two small meals, one around 11 am and one around 5 pm.

Alternate day fasting is perfect for losing weight for most people, but if you suffer from any congenital disease, I recommend contacting your doctor.

Spontaneous Meal Skipping

Spontaneous meal skipping is one of the easiest methods of intermittent Fasting; many people do it without even realizing it. For example, do you remember when you were teenagers and skipped a meal because you woke up too late on the weekend? Spontaneous meal skipping is practically skipping a meal now and then when you get the chance.

This method is ideal, especially for beginners who are approaching intermittent Fasting for the first time. My advice is to start by skipping a couple of meals a week and eventually increase to three or four. During this process, it is essential to pay attention to our body; spontaneous meal skipping is one of the IF methods with fewer side effects, but the risk of feeling tired or edgy exists. The best ways to avoid any side effects are to focus on a healthy and balanced diet and avoid skipping meals that are too close together. For example, I strongly advise against skipping two consecutive meals when using this method.

CHAPTER 3: HEALTH BENEFITS OF INTERMITTENT FASTING

Until now, you must have realized that intermittent fasting is simply switching between fasting and eating. Eating is done in cycles or specific periods and fasting is followed. There are numerous benefits of intermittent fasting.

Weight Loss

Intermittent Fasting switches from periods of eating to periods of fasting. If you fast, naturally, your calorie intake will reduce, and it also helps you maintain your weight loss. It also prevents you from indulging in mindless eating. Whenever you eat something, your body converts the food into glucose and fat. It uses this glucose immediately and stores the fat for later use. When you skip a few meals, your body starts to reach into its internal stores of fat to provide energy. Also, most of the fat that you lose is from the abdominal region. If you want a flat tummy, then this is the perfect diet for you.

Tackles Diabetes

Diabetes is a significant threat on its own. It is also a primary indicator of the increase in risk factors of various cardiovascular diseases like heart attacks and strokes. When the glucose level increases alarmingly in the bloodstream, and there isn't enough insulin to process this glucose, it causes diabetes. When your body resists insulin, it becomes difficult to regulate insulin levels in the body. Intermittent Fasting reduces insulin sensitivity and helps tackle diabetes.

Sleep

Lack of sleep is one of the main causes of obesity. When your body doesn't get enough sleep, the internal mechanism of burning fat suffers. Intermittent Fasting regulates your sleep cycle and, in turn, makes your body effectively burn fats. A good sleep cycle has different physiological benefits—it makes you feel energetic and elevates your overall mood.

Resistance to Illnesses

Intermittent Fasting helps in the growth and regeneration of cells. Did you know that the human body has an internal mechanism that helps repair damaged cells? Intermittent Fasting helps kickstart this mechanism. It improves the overall functioning of all the cells in the body. So, it is directly responsible for improving your body's natural defense mechanism by increasing its resistance to diseases and illnesses.

A Healthy Heart

Intermittent Fasting assists in weight loss, and weight loss improves your cardiovascular health. A buildup of plaque in blood vessels is known as atherosclerosis. This is the primary cause of various cardiovascular diseases. The endothelium is the thin lining of blood vessels, and any dysfunction in it results in atherosclerosis. Obesity is the primary problem that plagues humanity and is also the main reason for the increase of plaque deposits in the blood vessels. Stress and inflammation also increase the severity of this problem. Intermittent Fasting tackles the buildup of fat and helps tackle obesity. So, all you need to do is follow the simple protocols of Intermittent Fasting to improve your overall health.

A Healthy Gut

There are several millions of microorganisms present in your digestive system. These microorganisms help improve the overall functioning of your digestive system and are known as the gut microbiome. Intermittent Fasting enhances the health of these microbiomes and improves your digestive health. A healthy digestive system helps in better absorption of food and improves the functioning of your stomach.

Reduces Inflammation

Whenever your body feels there is an internal problem, its natural defense is inflammation. It doesn't mean that all forms of inflammation are desirable. Inflammation can cause several serious health conditions like arthritis, atherosclerosis, and other neurodegenerative disorders.

Any inflammation of this nature is known as chronic inflammation and is quite painful. Chronic inflammation can restrict your body's movements too.

Promotes Cell Repair

When you fast, the cells in your body start the process of waste removal. Waste removal means the breaking down of all dysfunctional cells and proteins and is known as autophagy. Autophagy offers protection against several degenerative diseases like Alzheimer's and cancer. You don't like accumulating garbage in your home, do you? Similarly, your body must not hold onto any unnecessary toxins. Autophagy is the body's way of getting rid of all things useless.

Higher Concentration and Brain Power

When subjected to food scarcity for a long time, mammals, including humans, will start to experience a decrease in their organ size. One of these organs is the brain. While some organs return to their original size over time, others may be impacted over the long term.

The brain handles the basic cognitive function of the body. In order to function properly and get the needed nutrients, it needs to return to its original size. However, if the brain becomes too foggy, getting the needed food nutrients will be pretty difficult, which might lead to malnutrition and even be fatal. However, during a shorter period of food scarcity, the brain becomes hyperactive in its search for food as a mechanism for survival.

Excessive availability of food and eating altogether makes us mentally dull. Reflect on a time when you were completely satisfied after a big meal. After eating a massive plate of food, you will likely go into a "food coma" and curl up and sleep, or maybe just watch your favorite TV show on Netflix rather than get the motivation to go achieve your goals. Without a doubt, satisfaction from food makes man naturally lose the drive to pursue his goals, which ultimately leads to dulling the brain. With this in mind, know that when you fast, your cognitive abilities are quickened. This improves your mental keenness, allowing you to achieve your health-related goals as opposed to excessively feeding.

It should be established here that there is no scientific research to support the notion that intermittent fasting alters mental alertness negatively. Fasting will not affect your cognitive function, such as moods, mental alertness, reaction time, intention, and sleep in any bad way. On the contrary, these things get boosted during fasting.

Promotes Autophagy and Protects Neurons

This is one of the many wonderful benefits of intermittent fasting, which many people should look forward to. Fasting is amazing in that it keeps the brain's cells from degeneration. This is because fasting prevents neural death.

Besides, fasting also triggers the process of autophagy in the brain—autophagy is the process in which the body gets rid of damaged body cells and brings out new ones. When the body is full of healthy, active, and improved cells, it is strong and well-equipped to combat any diseases that might want to attack.

With autophagy, the risk of viral infection, as well as duplication of intracellular parasites, reduces drastically. This dramatically reduces intracellular pathogens, such as cancer cells. Besides, the brain and other body tissue cells are protected from abnormal growth, inflammation, and toxicity.

Reduced Risk of Depression

With intermittent fasting, there is an increase in the levels of a neurotransmitter called "neurotrophic factor." When the body is deficient in this brain-derived factor, it contributes to significant issues such as depression and other mood disorders. Hence, intermittent fasting is really helpful in improving mental alertness and enhancing mood, which ultimately leads to a reduced tendency to develop these conditions.

There are a couple of metabolic features that get triggered when we fast that improve brain health. This explains why people who practice intermittent fasting do have lower levels of inflammation, low blood sugar levels, and reduced oxidative stress.

There are also indications that intermittent fasting can keep the brain protected against the risk of stroke.

Fosters Immune Regulation

When you fast, part of the primary aim of the body is to keep the immune system healthy. This is why we encourage drinking a large quantity of water during the period of the intermittent fast, and afterward as well. Water can be spiced up with other detox agents that remove toxins from the digestive system and reduce the number of unhealthy gut microbes. Have in mind that the number of gut microbes present in the gastrointestinal tract is directly related to the immune system's function.

Intermittent fasting determines the number of inflammatory cytokines that the body has. Hence, it helps regulate the body's overall immune system. In the body, we have two significant cytokines that cause inflammation in the body: Interleukin-6 and Tumor Necrosis Factor Alpha. Fasting suppresses the release of these inflammatory pro-inflammatory cytokines.

Reduces the Risk of Chronic Disease

People living with chronic autoimmune diseases like Crohn's disease, colitis, rheumatoid arthritis, and systemic lupus will definitely see remarkable improvement with intermittent fasting. The idea is simple. Fasting reduces the rate of an extreme inflammatory process in the bodies of these persons. With this, they have an ideal immune function.

For instance, cancer cells have between ten and seventy extra insulin receptors in contrast to healthy body cells. This happens as a result of the breakdown of sugar for fuel. With intermittent fasting, cancer cells are starved of sugar intake. This conditions the cells for damage through free radicals.

Improves Genetic Repair Mechanisms

The tendency of the body to live longer increases when it does not get enough food. This is because, with intermittent fasting, there is repair and regeneration of cells that come about via a repair mechanism in the body. This is understandable, as the energy required for cell repair is lesser when compared to what is necessary for cell creation or division.

Hence, during the period of intermittent fasting, cell division, and creation in the body becomes reduced. This is a necessary process, vital especially for the healing of malignant cells, which thrive as a result of abnormal cell division.

In the body, the human growth hormone (HGH) takes care of the process of cell repair. It is a human growth hormone that brings out changes in metabolism that cause tissue repair and fat burning. Thus, when we fast, the body can concentrate more on repairing body tissues with amino acids and enzymes. This restores tissue collagen and also triggers an improvement in bones, ligaments, tendons, and general muscle function in the body.

Reduce the Likelihood of Developing Cancer

Lastly, studies have found that intermittent fasting can reduce your likelihood of developing cancer and help make treatment more successful. As you are aware, intermittent fasting can help treat oxidative stress and cellular damage, both of which cause cancer. By reducing this damage, you can thereby reduce your risk of developing cancer in the future.

But that is not all. While human studies still need to be conducted, a study on mice found that when practicing short-term fasting, chemotherapy treatment becomes more successful in targeting and treating both breast cancer and skin cancer. Not only did the chemotherapy itself become more effective, but the mice's immune systems also were better able to fight off the cancerous cells and growths, which is essential as chemotherapy is well-known for reducing a person's immune system drastically.

CHAPTER 4: BEST WAY TO DO IT IN MENOPAUSE

Menopause is one of the most complicated phases in a woman's life. The time when our bodies begin to change and important natural transitions occur that are too often negatively affected, while it is important to learn how to change our eating habits and eating patterns appropriately. In fact, it often happens that a woman is not ready for this new condition and experiences it with a feeling of defeat as an inevitable sign of time travel, and this feeling of prostration turns out to be too invasive and involves many aspects of one's stomach.

It is therefore important to remain calm as soon as there are messages about the first signs of change in our human body, to ward off the onset of menopause for the right purpose and to minimize the negative effects of suffering, especially in the early days. Even during this difficult transition, targeted nutrition can be very beneficial.

What Happens to the Body of a Menopausal Woman?

It must be said that a balanced diet does not produce major weight fluctuations. This will no doubt be a factor that supports women who are going through menopause, but it is not a sufficient condition to present with classic symptoms that are felt, which can be classified according to the period experienced. In fact, we can distinguish between the pre-menopausal phase, which affects between 45 and 50 years, and is physiologically compatible with a drastic reduction in the production of the hormone estrogen (responsible for the menstrual cycle, which actually starts irregularly). This period is accompanied by a series of complex and highly subjective endocrine changes.

When someone enters actual menopause, estrogen hormone production decreases even more dramatically, the range of the symptoms widens, leading to large amounts of the hormone, for example, to a certain class called catecholamine adrenaline. The result of these changes is a dangerous heat wave, increased sweating, and the presence of tachycardia, which can be more or less severe.

However, the changes also affect the female genital organs, with the volume of the breasts, uterus and ovaries decreasing. The mucous membranes become less active and vaginal dryness increases. There may also be changes in bone balance, with decreased calcium intake and increased mobilization at the expense of the skeletal system. Because of this, there is a lack of continuous bone formation, and conversely, erosion begins, which is a predisposition for osteoporosis.

Although menopause causes major changes that greatly change a woman's body and soul, metabolism is one of the worst. In fact, during menopause, the absorption and accumulation of sugars and triglycerides changes and it is easy to increase some clinical values such as cholesterol and triglycerides, which lead to high blood pressure or arteriosclerosis. In addition, many women often complain of disturbing circulatory disorders and local edema, especially in the stomach. It also makes weight gain easier, even though you haven't changed your eating habits.

The Ideal Diet for Menopause

In cases where disorders related to the arrival of menopause become difficult to manage, drug or natural therapy under medical supervision may be necessary. The contribution given by a correct diet at this time can be considerable, in fact, given the profound variables that come into play, it is necessary to modify our food routine, both in order not to be surprised by all these changes, and to adapt in the most natural way possible.

The problem of fat accumulation in the abdominal area is always caused by the drop-in estrogen. In fact, they are also responsible for the classic hourglass shape of most women, which consists in depositing fat mainly on the hips, which begins to fail with menopause. As a result, we go from a gynoid condition to an android one, with an adipose increase localized on the belly. In addition, the metabolic rate of disposal is reduced, which means that even if you do not change your diet and eat the same quantities of food as you always have, you could experience weight gain, which will be more marked in the presence of bad habits or irregular diet.

The digestion is also slower and intestinal function becomes more complicated. This further contributes to swelling as well as the occurrence of intolerance and digestive disorders which have never been disturbed before. Therefore, the beginning will be more problematic and difficult to manage during this period. The distribution of nutrients must be different: reducing the amount of low carbohydrate, which is always preferred not to be purified, helps avoid the peak of insulin and at the same time maintains stable blood sugar.

Furthermore, it will be necessary to slightly increase the quantity of both animal and vegetable proteins; choose good fats, prefer seeds and extra virgin olive oil and severely limit saturated fatty acids (those of animal origin such as lard, lard, etc.). All this is to try to increase the proportion of antioxidants taken, which will help to counteract the effect of free radicals, whose concentration begins to increase during this period. It will be necessary to prefer foods rich in phytoestrogens, which will help to control the states of stress to which the body is subjected and which will favor, at least in part, the overall estrogenic balance.

These molecules are divided into three main groups and the foods that contain them should never be missing on our tables: isoflavones, present mainly in legumes such as soy and red clover; lignans, of which flax seeds and oily seeds, in general, are particularly rich; cumestani, found in sunflower seeds, beans and sprouts. The Calcium supplementation will be necessary through cheeses such as parmesan; dairy products such as yogurt, egg yolk, some vegetables such as rocket, Brussels sprouts, broccoli, spinach, asparagus; legumes; dried fruit such as nuts, almonds or dried grapes.

Excellent additional habits that will help to regain well-being may be: limiting sweets to sporadic occasions, thus drastically reducing sugars (for example by giving up sugar in coffee and getting used to drinking it bitterly); learning how to dose alcohol a lot (avoiding spirits, liqueurs and aperitif drinks) and choose only one glass of good wine when you are in company, this because it tends to increase visceral fat which is precisely what is going to settle at the level abdominal. Clearly, even by eating lots of fruit, it is difficult to reach a high carbohydrate quota as in a traditional diet. However, a dietary plan to follow can be useful to have a more precise indication of how to distribute the foods. Obviously, one's diet must be structured in a personal way, based on specific metabolic needs and one's lifestyle.

CHAPTER 5: FOODS TO CONSUME AND THOSE TO AVOID

No matter how you plot your path when it comes to an intermittent fast, you need to have an understanding of what is good to eat, and not to eat during your efforts. Unless you are engaging in a complete fast from solid foods for 24 hours, you will have to know just what you should eat on your fast days. Likewise, it would be good to know what might be best suited for your non-fast days too. Because remember, just because you might be on one of your non-fast days, doesn't mean it would be a good idea to go downtown and binge at all you can eat buffet. Here in this chapter, we will help guide you to make wise food choices on what to eat and what not to eat during your intermittent fasting.

What to Eat

Berries

Berries are very healthy, incredibly flavorful, and much lower in calories and sugar than you might think! Their tart sweetness can bring a smoothie to life, and they make a delicious snack on their own without any help from things like cream or sugar.

Cruciferous Vegetables

These are vegetables like cabbage, Brussels sprouts, broccoli, and cauliflower. These are beautiful additions to your diet because they're packed with vital nutrients and with fiber that your body will love and use quickly!

Eggs

Eggs are such a great addition to your diet because they're packed to the gills with protein, you can do just about anything with them, they're easy to prepare, travel well if you hard boil them, and they can pair with just about anything. They're an excellent protein source for salads, and they're right on their own as well.

Fish

In particular, whitefish is typically very lean, but fish like salmon that have a little bit of color in them are packed with protein, fats, and oils that are great for you. They're good for brain and heart health, and there's a massive array of delicious things you can do with them.

Healthy Starches Like Individual Potatoes (With Skins!)

In particular, red potatoes are excellent to eat, even if you're trying to lose weight because your body can use those carbs for fuel, and the skins are packed with minerals that your body will enjoy. A little bit of potato here and there can-do good things for your nutrition, but they are also a great way to feel like you're getting a little more of those fun foods that you should cut back on.

Legumes

Beans, beans, the magical fruit. They're packed with protein, and the starch in them makes them stick to your ribs without making you pay for it later. They're lovely in soups, salads, and just about any other meal of the day that you're looking to fill out. By adding beans to your regimen, you might find that your meals stick with you a little bit longer and leave you feeling more satisfied than you thought possible.

Nuts

I know you've heard people talking about how a handful of almonds makes a great snack, and if you're anything like me, you've always had kind of a hard time believing it. Nuts, as it turns out, have a good deal of their healthy fats in them that your body can use to get through those rough patches and, while they were not the most satisfying snack on their own, you might consider topping your salad with them for a little bit of crunch, or pairing them with some berries to make them a little more satisfying.

Probiotics Help Boost Your Gut Health

Having a happy gut often means that your dietary success and overall health will improve!

Vegetables That Are Rich in Healthy Fats

Not to sound topical or trendy, but avocados are a great example of a vegetable packed with healthy fats. Look for vegetables with fatty acids and a higher fat content, and you will find that if you add more of those into your regimen, you will get hungry less often.

Water, Water, Water, and More Water

No matter what you decide to add to or subtract from your regimen, stay hydrated. It will help digestive health and ease, and it will keep you from feeling down or tired, keeping you from getting too hungry. Add electrolytes where you need to, and don't be shy about bringing a bottle with you when you go from place to place. Stay hydrated!

What to Avoid

Grains

Whole grains may have their health benefits and be full of fiber, and you can also get these nutrients elsewhere. The human diet does not require grain consumption. The truth is while grains may have some benefits, they are ridiculously high in both total and net carbohydrates, making them incompatible with the ketogenic diet.

Some people do try what is known as the targeted ketogenic diet, which is a version of the diet specifically designed for those who complete extended and strenuous workouts. With the targeted ketogenic diet, a person will consume a small serving of carb-heavy food, such as grains, for thirty to forty minutes before working out.

Starchy Vegetables and Legumes

Some vegetables are high in carbohydrates. It includes potatoes, beans, beets, corn, and more. These vegetables may have nutritional benefits, but you can get these same nutrients in low-carb vegetable alternatives.

Sugary Fruits

Most fruits contain a high sugar content, meaning that they are also high in carbohydrates. It is important to avoid most fruits. The exception is that you can enjoy berries, lemons, and limes in moderation. Some people will also enjoy a small serving of melon as a treat from time to time, but watch your portion size as it can add up quickly!

Milk and Low-Fat Dairy Products

As you can enjoy dairy products such as cheese on the ketogenic diet, sadly, milk is much higher in carbohydrates than cheese, with a glass of two-percent milk containing twelve carbs, half of your daily total. Instead, choose low-carb and dairy-free milk alternatives such as almond, coconut, and soy milk.

You may consider using low-fat cheeses instead of full fat to reduce the saturated fats you are consuming. The reason for this is that when the cheese is made with low-fat dairy, it naturally has a higher carbohydrate content, which will cut into your daily net carb total.

Cashews, Pistachios, and Chestnuts

While you can enjoy nuts and seeds in moderation, keep in mind that nuts contain a significant level of carbohydrates and therefore should be eaten with caution.

If you want to enjoy nuts, you can fully enjoy almonds, pecans, walnuts, macadamia nuts, and other options instead of these options.

Most Natural Sweeteners

While you can undoubtedly enjoy sugar-free natural sweeteners such as stevia, monk fruit, and sugar alcohols, you should avoid natural sweeteners that contain sugar. Suffice to say, the sugar content makes these sweeteners naturally high in carbs. But not only that, but they will also spike your blood sugar and insulin. It means you should avoid things such as honey, agave, maple, coconut palm sugar, and dates.

Alcohol

Alcohol is not generally enjoyed on the ketogenic diet, as your body will be unable to burn off calories while your liver attempts to process alcohol. Many people also find that when they are in ketosis, they get drunk more quickly and experience more severe hangovers. Not only that, but alcohol adds unnecessary calories and carbohydrates to your diet.

The worst offenders to choose would be margaritas, piña coladas, sangrias, Bloody Mary, whiskey sours, cosmopolitans, and regular beers.

But, if you choose to drink alcohol do so in moderation and choose low-carb versions such as rum, vodka, tequila, whiskey, and gin. The next-best options would be dry wines and light beers.

CHAPTER 6: MISTAKES TO AVOID

Intermittent Fasting is a great process that can bring exemplary health effects. However, any process can only work efficiently if its execution is right, and silly mistakes are not made in it.

This chapter will explain some of the common mistakes women make while following intermittent fasting. This chapter will focus on the basic mistakes that we make casually but which can harm our weight loss goals as well as health goals drastically.

Going All-in

Perhaps the most common mistake is going "all-in" right away. By this, we mean that you set out to do a 10-hour fast, for instance, at the drop of a hat. This is not only counterproductive but also downright dangerous.

You see, when you make the decision to take up intermittent fasting, you need to ease your way into it. You can't just expect to go without food straight away. If you do this, you could put your health at serious risk. The most common symptoms include irritability, dizziness, and even anxiety.

So, the solution to this situation is to ease into intermittent fasting. The best way is to gradually spread yourself out so that you can confidently start out with an 8-hour fast. If you are sleeping a full 8 hours regularly, all you need to do is make sure that you don't consume any food at least an hour before bedtime. Then, try your best to avoid consuming any food until at least 30 minutes after rising.

Please make sure to pace yourself to avoid the most unpleasant symptoms that come when you go too long without food.

Binging Before and After Fasting

A common mistake is having a big meal right before a fast. The logic here is that you are "stocking up" for the time you won't be eating. That is not only a mistake, but it's also counterproductive. When you do this, your body goes out of whack. It might think that there is something wrong and may choose to hoard calories instead of burning them off.

By the same token, binging after a fasting day is a one-way ticket to digestive distress. After a short, it's still a good idea to eat something light. That way, you can give your metabolism and digestive system a chance to adjust to food again. The longer you go without food, the easier you need to take it on your digestive system.

Fasting Too Often

Those intermittent fasting practitioners that believe that "more is better" are only asking for trouble. When you fast too often, your body may enter starvation mode. This means that the body thinks that something is going on, and food is scarce. So rather than use up fat stores, the body begins to hoard as much as it can. This is where intermittent fasting practitioners plateau and subsequently begin gaining weight.

This is why the recommended guideline is to fast two times a week, three times tops. Ideally, you would leave at least a couple of days in between fasts. If you are able to accustom your body to consume less food, then your body won't think that there is something wrong when you fast. It will simply draw on its stores. In this manner, you can avoid triggering starvation mode.

Not Fasting Enough

While this isn't a mistake per se, it is simply not the most efficient practice. Not fasting enough means fasting once or twice a month. Please note that 24-hour fasts, the ones which are recommended once a month, are fasts that are done in addition to regular fast days. Consequently, it's best to have a regular routine. This will allow your body to find a rhythm that will ensure that you get the most out of your intermittent fasting practice.

Additionally, please try to avoid an irregular routine. For instance, you decide to fast for three days a week over four weeks, and then go weeks without fasting. What this will do is throw your body out of whack. When the body is out of whack, it will naturally resort to starvation mode. Moreover, you may end up experiencing some of the most unpleasant symptoms that come when you don't eat. So, this is why we advocate having a regular routine as much as possible.

Falling Into a Predictable Routine

While routines are important, the body may also fall into a predictable rut if you maintain the same routine for too long. When the body eventually gets used to the new routine, you may find that you plateau in your weight loss goals. To avoid this, it's important to shake things up a bit.

The most effective way that intermittent fasting practitioners shake off falling into a routine is by switching up their approach. For instance, some folks like to start off with the 5:2 methods. Then, after a three or four-month period, switch to an alternating day fast. After the other three or four months, they switch over to the time-restricted method. Once they achieve a high level of proficiency, they may choose to throw in a 24-hour fast every so often.

Pay Attention to Macronutrients

This is one of the most important things to remember. The people who are suffering from obesity simply want to get rid of this malice. They are ready to barter anything for it. They dream of a slender figure as the ultimate goal, and this is where they become susceptible to making some of the most fatal mistakes.

Intermittent fasting or any form of dieting or calorie-restrictive routine would put certain restrictions on you. Intermittent fasting doesn't put a cap on the amount of food you can eat or its type. However, that doesn't mean you can eat a lot. In most cases, you will have only 7-8 hours in reality to eat anything that you want. While it can seem to take a long time, the time for the last meal of the day approaches much sooner than the previous meal has been digested. Missing that meal may mean that you'll have to go without food till the next meal. Therefore, the amount of food you can eat gets limited.

Don't Get Greedy in the Fasting Windows

Food has its own temptation. It looks like the most alluring thing in the world when you have been deprived of it for a long time. This would happen to you too. But you mustn't get greedy at such times and lose control. You must properly get off your fasting windows.

The most common blunder people make is overeating after they've broken their fast. This can cause several problems, and poor digestion is one of them. In the fasting state, the gut gets to stay away from food for extended periods, and hence it can get a bit dry. Stuffing it with heavy food can cause problems. Starting with liquid food and progressing to semi-solid and solid foods is the perfect way to start the day.

Don't Try to Rush the Process

Slow and steady wins the race. This is an adage we all have heard, but most of us fail to believe it. We want quick results, and for that, we are ready to make the jumps. However, this is not how the body works. Your body makes the transition very slowly. It needs the time to adjust to any kind of change, positive or negative, and the same would happen even in the case of intermittent fasting.

If you want to succeed with the process, you must ensure that you stick to every stage for some time. You must give your body the required time to adjust. There would be decades-old habits that would need to change, and it can be difficult for your body at times. You must not hurry the process if you want your body to respond positively to the transition.

Perseverance Is the Key

Impatience is a big problem in people battling with weight. There is no fault of theirs as they are already under great pressure. Most people trying to lose weight have already faced disappointment with other weight loss measures, and hence they want to see the results fast to believe them. They are not ready to wait very long to get the results.

This is a point where problems can occur. Intermittent fasting is not any wonder process. It is a wonderful process, but it doesn't work by magic. It tries to correct the problems that may have reached their current state of development in decades, at least.

Don't Frame Unrealistic Expectations

We all like to dream big, and that is a good thing. However, we must also remain grounded in reality. This will help in accepting the facts and save a lot of disappointments. Many times, we are so engrossed with imaginary expectations that we fail to recognize the gifts we get. If weight loss is your target, consider how much time you're willing to spend, how much you're willing to go, and any medical problems you're dealing with. Without considering all these facts, expecting a complete makeover would be absurd. If you have made such expectations, then you will not even be able to enjoy the weight loss you are observing. Your expectations would overshadow the results. You must remain realistic.

CHAPTER 7: TIPS AND TRICKS

Before you begin fasting, there are some things that you will want to do to prepare yourself. It may be difficult mentally and physically, especially if you are new to fasting. Your mindset will become very important as you are fasting, especially the longer you fast at one time.

Ensure You Are Fasting in a Healthy Way

When it comes to fasting, it is important to ensure that you approach it in a way that will be beneficial for your health, and that will not do more harm than good.

Firstly, you want to maintain flexibility with yourself and your body when fasting. If you are not feeling well as you are trying to fast, don't be afraid to eat a small amount on your fast days. This is especially true at the beginning when you first introduce fasting into your diet. If you try a water fast for example, and you feel lightheaded and weak, you may decide that you want to instead try an intermittent fasting method like 5:2 which would allow you to eat on your fast days, but in a greatly restricted amount.

Obtain Proper Nutrition and Rest

Sleeping is an essential part of human life, and getting the amount of sleep a body needs to run well will help you in intermittent fasting, keeping you active.

If you're attempting 24-hour water fast, make sure that the last meal of your day is eaten well before bedtime. Eat something nutritious (not overly full of fat and carbohydrates) and drink a large amount of water during the hour leading up to bedtime so that when hunger begins to set in, there are enough nutrients in your body to keep you going for at least three or four hours.

If you're attempting a multi-day fast or one in which you'll be fasting while walking or working outside, make sure to eat plenty of fruits when they're in season and take the time to schedule breaks for food and rest. If you feel light-headed or weak from hunger, take the time to sit down and eat something so that you aren't forced to stop the fast for a meal. Fasting should never be exhausting or uncomfortable, so make certain that you're getting enough of what your body needs during the day so that it's easy to continue.

Making massive changes in your diet or attempting things like fasting too soon before going on vacation can be very stressful and detrimental to your overall health, so don't rush it. Focus on eating healthier foods over time instead of drastically changing your routine right away.

When you're eating every other day, don't be afraid of trying new foods or preparing meals in different ways. You deserve a break from the same old foods that you've been eating for years. Don't be afraid to approach your food planning differently than you normally would, and don't forget to enjoy it!

Add Some Exercise

If possible, try to do some form of exercise before beginning your first fast so that your body is prepared for what lies ahead. Whether you work out during the week or not, you're going to be burning far more calories than normal while fasting and it would be a good idea to prepare your body in some way.

Just a few minutes each day are enough, to begin with, and as you get used to doing so, you can increase the length of your workouts until you feel at optimal health. This way, when you do fast, your body doesn't experience any loss of energy and is able to keep up its normal functions.

Walking is an excellent form of exercise for weight loss that doesn't require any special equipment or training. You can also try doing some aerobic exercises during the weekend if you're accustomed to working out at this time.

When it comes to the weight loss benefits of fasting, there's no shortage of information, and studies have proven that a prolonged period of fasting can lead to a significant weight loss.

The only thing you'll need is a dehydrator and some food – yes, you can still go through the process of fasting even if you're at work! You just need to make sure you always have snacks with you so that your body won't get too hungry all the time. You will also need to know when you should drink water, as well as what kinds of foods you should and shouldn't consume.

Always remember to eat breakfast, snack on protein-rich foods throughout the day, get a good night's sleep and drink a lot of water. This isn't too hard and will help you not only look skinny but also be healthy. There are many ways for you to lose weight rapidly, but the best method is through dieting and exercising properly.

Increase Your Water Intake

Dehydration can accompany fasting since much of our water intake throughout the day comes from the food we eat, like fruits or vegetables. If you are feeling like you are dehydrated while fasting (dry mouth, headache), it is important to increase your water intake. You will also want to ensure you drink enough water each time you fast afterward. The recommendation is about two liters per day, but of course, this depends on your body size. In general, eight glasses of water that are about eight ounces each should give you enough water to be hydrated but when fasting, this must increase to about nine to thirteen glasses. This works out to be between two and three liters of water.

Pay Attention to Your Body

If you are feeling very unwell while you are fasting, it is important to know when to stop fasting. It is normal to feel fatigued, hungry, and maybe irritable when you fast, but you may want to stop your fast if you feel completely unwell. In order to be safe, for your first few times fasting, keep the duration shorter, and work your way up to the desired amount of time. Also, keep some food on you in case you need to eat something due to low blood sugar or feeling unwell. Remember that you are fasting to take care of your body and your health and it should not make you feel worse.

Avoid Stress

Whenever we began something new, especially if it is related to our body, we need to consider the possible stress it may cause. Stressing out about it might make it worst. Keep calm, do your thing, and do not stress out. Remember that fasting implies not eating foods for some time. When fasting, be consistent with yourself and try not to eat before the named time. It will guarantee that you lose the greatest amount of weight and get the most benefits from intermittent fasting in solid terms.

Increase Protein Intake

Ensuring that you eat enough protein while fasting will have numerous benefits for you. Protein takes longer to digest, which means that the energy you get from protein will be longer lasting than the energy you get from other sources like carbohydrates- which is used up quite quickly. This will keep you from having an energy "crash" similar to a sugar crash after you have quickly used up the sugars you have ingested.

Select the Foods You Eat Wisely

When you do break your fast or when you are eating small amounts on fasting days, choose the foods you eat wisely. You want to properly prepare your body to fast and keep it healthy while you do so. In addition to eating enough protein, you want to make sure that the other foods you eat are real, whole foods. Whole foods are those which are as close to those found in nature as possible. These are things like meats, vegetables, fruits, fish, eggs, and legumes. This will give you all of the nutrients you need to stay healthy. Eating fast food and processed foods on the days that you are not fasting will leave you feeling tired and without energy, especially if you are fasting the next day or have fasted the day before.

Consider Supplementation

Supplementing may be very beneficial and even necessary when fasting to maintain and improve health. Some essential nutrients and minerals that your body would greatly benefit from like Omega-3's or iron may be difficult to get in adequate amounts if you are fasting. For this reason, supplementing them may benefit you in terms of keeping you feeling healthy and energetic, as well as keeping your brain functioning to its full potential. You can take specific nutrients on their own in pill form or you can opt for a multivitamin that will include all of the most essential vitamins and minerals for overall good health. The vitamins included in a multivitamin will be those that are known to promote good overall health and those that are usually obtained through a balanced, whole food diet.

Avoid Overdoing It in the Beginning

Keeping your exercise levels to a minimum while fasting is often necessary as your body will not have as many readily-available sugars or carbohydrates to provide you with the quick energy needed for a workout. This is especially important if you are beginning a fasting regimen for the first time. If you are planning to increase your levels of autophagy through a combination of fasting and exercise, wait until your body has adapted to your fasting routine before adding in the exercise portion of the plan.

Find Something to Do When You Fast

It is said that an inactive mind is the devil's showroom. When you fast intermittently and are not busy, food will be the only thing on your mind, compelling you to eat before the fast-breaking time. You can learn a new skill or get a hobby, start reading or research about anything that interests you.

Detoxify your Body

Your body is a magnificent piece of creative magic that was built to operate for the entire length of your life on earth. It is made up of a number of complex systems, each of which has a vital role to play in sustaining your life. When any one of these systems is compromised in any way, the negative knock-on effect for the entire body can be devastating.

As you age, inflammation often becomes a challenge. Start by taking stock of the type of food you are currently eating that may be causing inflammation. Plan your diet to exclude as many of these foods as possible:

Refined sugar: This is found in cakes, candy, sugar, and desserts.
Refined carbohydrates: This is found in bread, pasta, pastries, and cookies.
Processed meats: Some are ham, salami, bacon, and jerky
Foods with MSG: Some foods are instant noodles, instant mash, etc.
Artificial trans-fats: This can be found in certain margarine, French fries, fast foods, microwave popcorn, etc.
Alcohol.
Vegetable and seed oils: Some include soy, sunflower seed oil, etc.

Include a wide variety of anti-inflammatory foods such as broccoli, fresh vegetables, fruits, lean meat, fish, and lots of water.

CHAPTER 8: FAQ

Is the Intermittent Fasting Diet a Good Option for Me?

So, does an intermittent fasting diet work when compared to other diets? The answer here is a resounding yes. For example, using a 16 hour fast will keep your body burning fat for most of every day! And getting all of your calories during a relatively small eating window stops your body from going into starvation mode and desperately hanging onto body fat. Compared to a regular reduced-calorie diet, this is a huge difference. While any reduced-calorie approach will initially lead to fat loss, your body is an efficient machine. It will compensate by slowing down your metabolism (the exact opposite of what you want) and holding onto body fat.

Is the Intermittent Fasting Diet Restrictive?

Any diet, by its very nature, involves making better food choices. If someone tries to sell you on the pancake diet, run a mile! Eating rubbish can never be a good choice. However, most diets will have you try to eat clean all the time. It is tough to do and is directly linked to finding yourself eating 12 doughnuts in one sitting after a couple of weeks of deprivation! Intermittent fasting also involves healthy food choices, but it does give you more wiggle room. It is difficult to overeat junk in a small eating window after you have already had your healthy food. It does let you eat enough to stop you from falling off the wagon, however.

Perhaps the real advantage of intermittent fasting is that it can be a lifestyle rather than a short-term approach. With most diets, even if you do manage to follow it long enough to get results to be followed by a rebound-that, it is a return to poor eating and fat gain. By viewing fasting as a long-term solution, this problem effectively disappears.

Should I Take Vitamins When I Intermittently Fast?

It is more important than ever to take vitamins and supplements when fasting, as you are skipping meals that were helping to supply you with these vital nutrients, and you must replace them. The biggest problem with vitamins and fasting is that taking a vitamin pill in a fasted state may result in stomach pain, nausea, and diarrhea. To avoid these unpleasant, unsettling effects, try and get your vitamins down while in the fed state. If this is impossible, try taking your vitamins at night so you can sleep through the discomfort.

Alternatively, you might choose vitamins in liquid form, as they are easier to digest while fasting. If you don't usually take vitamins, a basic multivitamin that provides 100% of your daily intake is a great start to ensure you aren't missing out on anything while intermittently fasting.

Why Would Anyone Fast Who Doesn't Want to Lose Weight?

It may seem odd to someone who is considering intermittently fasting to lose weight, for anyone who has their weight under control to change their eating habits or patterns. After all, aren't they already living the dream? Let's not forget about all the other benefits of intermittent fasting:

Fasting for health benefits: Some people swear by fasting because they feel it improves their sleep, mental clarity and helps them control and maintain chronic diseases such as diabetes, cardiovascular disease, multiple sclerosis, fibromyalgia, chronic fatigue syndrome, cancer, and the side effects from chemotherapy.

Fasting for athletes: Fasting offers a consistent method of fueling and resting the body that works under many of the same principles as training and rest days. It provides them a much more convenient way to ensure that they consume the food they need to train than the other option of eating small meals every 2 or 3 hours. It allows them to maintain a nutrition routine that provides a lengthier feeding time which can be enjoyed with friends and family.

Fasting for busy people with poor eating habits: People who travel a lot for business often feel less than well most of the time due to poor eating habits developed due to airport restaurants and late-night vending machines.

Make sure you are well-hydrated and avoid salty or sugary foods before you fast.

Don't stuff yourself the night before your fast. This "last supper" mentality is a rookie mistake that will give you indigestion, a poor night's sleep, and an even ruder awakening to your stomach and brain when you follow up the preceding evening's bacchanalia with a fasting period.

Why Do I Get Headaches When I Fast, and How Can I Stop Them?

Complaints of headaches, especially when beginning an intermittent fasting program, are pretty standard. If you are waking with a headache, you may not have hydrated yourself enough the night before. Not drinking enough water is one of the biggest culprits of headaches during fasting, and water should be imbibed throughout the fasting/feeding process. Headaches can also be a side effect of the detoxing process that occurs in intermittent fasting. They will be especially prevalent in the beginning stages of incorporating the program into your health regime.

Isn't Intermittent Fasting Just a Fancy Way of Saying I'm Starving Myself?

Fatty acids are used by the body as an energy source for muscles but lower the amount of glucose that travels to the brain. Fatty acids also include a chemical called glycerol that can be used, like glucose, as an energy source, but it too will eventually run out.

Fat stores are depleted, and the body turns to stored protein for energy, breaking down muscle tissue. The muscle tissue breaks down very quickly. When all sources of protein are gone, cells can no longer function.

The body does not have the energy to fight off bacteria and viruses. It takes 8 to 12 weeks to starve to death, although there have been cases of people surviving 25 weeks or more.

Is Intermittent Fasting Safe for Women?

Women are more hormonally sensitive than men. Because of this, they may respond more intensely to the challenges of intermittent fasting and need to consult with a medical professional before starting a periodic fasting program, especially if they have menstrual and fertility issues. Once intermittent fasting has been undertaken, women should also pay special attention to their menstrual cycle and seek medical guidance if they begin missing periods.

There is a modified technique of intermittent fasting that will help women who experience hormonal sensitivity. It is a more progressive approach that will help the female body adapt to fasting.

Fast for 12-16 hours
On fasting days, stick to light workouts such as yoga or light cardio
Fast on 2-3 nonconsecutive days per week
After a few weeks, add another day of fasting and monitor how it goes.
Drink loads of water
Save strength training for feeding periods or feeding days.

Why Can't I Have a Protein Shake When I'm Fasting?

You can't eat food when you are intermittently fasting – hence you can't drink a protein shake. People get confused about protein shakes – check out diet, fitness, nutrition, and health websites if you don't believe me. I used to shake my head in wonder when I first saw this question asked.

If you are on a 5:2 type of intermittent fasting program and you are consuming 500 to 600 calories on your "low" days, feel free to indulge in one or 2 of these shakes if they don't bring you over your total calorie count. If you are on Whole Day Fasting or in the fasting portion of your Time-Restricted intermittent fasting cycle, don't even think about it!

How Can I Fast When I'm on Vacation?

I indirectly referred to the answer to this question when I explained some of the advantages of Whole Day Fasting and 5:2 Intermittent Fasting. Because you are confining your fasting to 2 nonconsecutive days of the week, you can automatically end up with a 4-day feeding unit time. It will help the eating challenges of holidays and vacations in a big way.

CHAPTER 9: MEAL PLAN FOR 30 DAYS

Day	11 PM – 7 AM	Meal 1	Meal 1	Meal 1	Dessert
1	Fasting	Egg Omelet	Pork Carnitas	Vegan Lentil Burger	Brazil Nut Cheese
2	Fasting	Cinnamon and Pecan Porridge	Zuppa Toscana with Cauliflower	Roasted Carrots and Cashew Salad on Lemon Vinaigrette	Zucchini Bread Pancakes
3	Fasting	Creamy Mango and Banana Overnight Oats	Butter Chicken	Roasted Broccoli with Lemon, Garlic and Toasted Pine Nuts	Peanut Butter Bars
4	Fasting	Cinnamon Porridge	Creamy Lamb Korma	Instant Pot Teriyaki Chicken	Homemade Protein Bar
5	Fasting	Awesome Oatmeal	Chinese Chicken Salad	Savory Oatmeal Bowl	Chocolate Crunch Bars
6	Fasting	Low Carb Pancake Crepes	Homemade Turkey Burger and Relish	Reds Salad on Bacon and Balsamic Vinaigrette	Shortbread Cookies
7	Fasting	Avocado Egg Bowls	Smoked Salmon and Avocado Stacks	Maple Walnut-Glazed Black-Eyed Peas with Collard Greens	Chocolate Mousse
8	Fasting	Chia Seed Banana Blueberry Delight	Bacon Egg and Sausage Cups	Chicken Tetrazzini	Baked Apples
9	Fasting	Buttery Date Pancakes	Chicken in Sweet and Sour Sauce with Corn Salad	Raspberry Jam and Peanut Butter Overnight Oats	Quinoa Porridge

10	Fasting	Savory Breakfast Muffins	Asparagus and Pistachios Vinaigrette	Mixed Vegetables and Chicken Egg Rolls	Pumpkin Ice Cream
11	Fasting	Morning Meatloaf	Pork Carnitas	Turmeric Tofu Scramble	Apple Quinoa
12	Fasting	Sesame-Seared Salmon	Teriyaki Salmon	Poached Eggs and Bacon on Toast	Blueberry Cupcakes
13	Fasting	Eggs and Salsa	Butternut Squash Risotto	Quick and Easy Squash Soup	Kamut Porridge
14	Fasting	Grapefruit Yogurt Parfait	Mini Thai Lamb Salad Bites	Meatloaf	Overnight "Oats"
15	Fasting	Wholesome Mushroom and Cauliflower Risotto	Sesame-Seared Salmon	Vegan Coconut Kefir Banana Muffins	Avocado Pudding
16	Fasting	Keto Oatmeal	Garlic Butter Beef Steak	Veggie-Stuffed Omelet	Apple Crisp
17	Fasting	Poached Egg	Instant Pot Teriyaki Chicken	Kale & Artichoke Soup	Apple Quinoa
18	Fasting	Green Pineapple	Cheesy Taco Skillet	Filipino Chicken Adobo	Berry Sorbet
19	Fasting	Bacon and Eggs with Tomatoes	Lamb Curry	Asparagus and Green Peas Salad	Chocolate Crunch Bars
20	Fasting	Cinnamon and Pecan Porridge	Salmon with Sauce	Sesame-Ginger Chicken Salad	Baked Apples
21	Fasting	Low Carb	Homemade	Instant Pot	Berry Sorbet

		Pancake Crepes	Turkey Burger and Relish	Teriyaki Chicken	
22	Fasting	Buttery Date Pancakes	Smoked Salmon and Avocado Stacks	Savory Oatmeal Bowl	Chocolate Mousse
23	Fasting	Cinnamon and Pecan Porridge	Bacon Egg and Sausage Cups	Reds Salad on Bacon and Balsamic Vinaigrette	Peanut Butter Bars
24	Fasting	Sesame-Seared Salmon	Zuppa Toscana with Cauliflower	Maple Walnut-Glazed Black-Eyed Peas with Collard Greens	Homemade Protein Bar
25	Fasting	Awesome Oatmeal	Butter Chicken	Vegan Lentil Burger	Quinoa Porridge
26	Fasting	Grapefruit Yogurt Parfait	Mini Thai Lamb Salad Bites	Roasted Carrots and Cashew Salad on Lemon Vinaigrette	Zucchini Bread Pancakes
27	Fasting	Eggs and Salsa	Sesame-Seared Salmon	Filipino Chicken Adobo	Overnight "Oats"
28	Fasting	Avocado Egg Bowls	Garlic Butter Beef Steak	Asparagus and Green Peas Salad	Blueberry Cupcakes
29	Fasting	Savory Breakfast Muffins	Cheesy Taco Skillet	Meatloaf	Brazil Nut Cheese
30	Fasting	Cinnamon Porridge	Lamb Curry	Vegan Coconut Kefir Banana Muffins	Shortbread Cookies

CHAPTER 10: BREAKFAST

---

1. Avocado Egg Bowls

Preparation Time: 5 minutes   **Cooking Time:** 25 minutes   **Servings:** 3

Ingredients:

- 1 tsp. coconut oil
- 2 organics eggs, free-range
- Salt and pepper
- 1 large & ripe avocado

For Garnishing:

- Chopped walnuts
- Balsamic Pearls
- Fresh thyme

Directions:

Slice your avocado in two, then take out the pit and remove enough of the inside so that there is enough space inside to accommodate an entire egg.

Cut off a little bit of the bottom of the avocado so that the avocado will sit upright as you place it on a stable surface.

Open your eggs and put each of the yolks in a separate bowl or container. Place the egg whites in the same small bowl. Sprinkle some pepper and salt into the whites, according to your personal taste, then mix them well.

Melt the coconut oil in a pan that has a lid that fits and put it on med-high.

Put in the avocado boats, with the meaty side down on the pan, the skin side up, and sauté them for approx. 35 seconds, or when they become darker in color.

Turn them over, then add to the spaces inside, almost filling the inside with the whites of the eggs. Then, reduce the temperature and place the lid. Let them sit covered for approx. 16 to 20 minutes until the whites are just about fully cooked.

Gently add 1 yolk onto each of the avocados and keep cooking them for 4 to 5 mins, just until they get to the point of cooking you want them at.

Move the avocados to a dish and add toppings to each of them using the walnuts, the balsamic pearls, or/and thyme.

Nutrition: Calories: 215; Fat: 18g; Carbs: 8g; Protein: 9g.

---

2. Buttery Date Pancakes

Preparation Time: 10 minutes   **Cooking Time:** 10 minutes   **Servings:** 3

Ingredients:

- ¼ cup almond flour
- 3 eggs, beaten
- 1 tsp. olive oil
- 6 dates, pitted
- 1 tbsp. almond butter
- 1 tsp. vanilla extract
- ½ tsp. ground cinnamon

Directions:

Stir the eggs in a bowl to make them fluffy.
Wash the dates and cut them in half.
Discard the seeds and mash them finely.
Melt the almond butter and add to the eggs.
Add the almond flour, olive oil and cinnamon.
Mix well and add the vanilla extract.
Mix into a smooth batter.
Add the date paste and mix well.
In a pan heat the butter over medium heat.
Add the butter using a spoon and fry them golden brown from both sides.
Repeat with all the batter.
Serve with melted butter on top.

Nutrition: Calories: 281; Fat: 20g; Protein: 10.5g; Carbs: 4.5g.

3. Low Carb Pancake Crepes

Preparation Time: 10 minutes   **Cooking Time:** 10 minutes   **Servings:** 2

Ingredients:

- 3 oz. cream cheese
- 1 tsp. ground cinnamon
- 1 tbsp. honey
- 1 tsp. ground cardamom
- 1 tsp. butter
- 2 eggs, beaten

Directions:

In a bowl, whisk the eggs finely.
Beat the cream cheese in a different bowl until it becomes soft. batter
Add the egg mixture to the softened cream cheese and mix well until there are no lumps left.
Add cinnamon, cardamom, and honey to it. Mix well. The batter would be runnier than the pancake batter.
In a pan add the butter and heat over medium heat.
Add the batter using a scooper, that way all the sizes of the crepes would be the same.
Fry them golden brown on both sides.
Repeat the process with the rest of the batter.
Drizzle some honey on top and enjoy.

Nutrition: Calories: 241; Fat: 21.8g; Carbs: 2.4g; Protein: 9.6g.

4. Chia Seed Banana Blueberry Delight

Preparation Time: 30 minutes   **Cooking Time:** 0 minutes   **Servings:** 2

Ingredients:

- 1 cup yogurt
- ½ cup blueberries
- ½ tsp. Salt
- ½ tsp. Cinnamon
- 1 banana
- 1 tsp. Vanilla Extract
- ¼ cup Chia Seeds

Directions:

Discard the skin of the banana.
Cut into semi-thick circles.
You can mash them or keep them as a whole if you like to bite into your fruits.
Clean the blueberries properly and rinse well.
Soak the chia seeds in water for 30 minutes or longer.
Drain the chia seeds and transfer them into a bowl.
Add the yogurt and mix well.
Add the salt, cinnamon, and vanilla and mix again.
Now fold in the bananas and blueberries gently.
If you want to add dried fruit or nuts, add them and then serve immediately.
This is best served cold.

Nutrition: Calories: 260; Fat: 26.6g; Carbs: 17.4g; Protein: 4.1g.

5. Egg Omelet

Preparation Time: 10 minutes   **Cooking Time:** 10 minutes   **Servings:** 2

Ingredients:

- 1 cup cherry tomatoes
- 2 sausages, cooked
- 1 cup spinach
- ½ tsp. oregano
- Salt to taste
- Pepper to taste
- 2 eggs
- 2 tbsps. heavy cream

Directions:

Finely chop the cherry tomatoes.
Cut off the stem of the spinach. Chop them finely.
Crumble the sausage using your hands.
Mix the eggs with heavy cream in a bowl and add to the skillet.
Top the egg with cherry tomatoes, spinach, oregano and sausage.
Season using pepper and salt
Fold the omelet carefully.
Serve with more oregano on top.

Nutrition: Calories: 289; Fat: 53.9g; Carbs: 7.9g; Protein: 19.3g.

6. Savory Breakfast Muffins

Preparation Time: 10 minutes   **Cooking Time:** 25 minutes   **Servings:** 6

Ingredients:

- 8 eggs
- 1 cup shredded cheese
- Salt and pepper to taste
- ½ tsp. baking powder
- ¼ cup diced onion
- ⅔ cup coconut flour
- 1½ cup spinach
- ¼ cup full fat coconut milk
- 1 tbsp. basil, chopped
- ½ cup cooked chicken, diced finely

Directions:

Preheat the oven to 375°F.
Use butter or oil to grease your muffin tray or you can use muffin paper liners.
In a large mixing bowl, whisk the eggs.
Add in the coconut milk and mix again.
Gradually shift in the coconut flour with baking powder and salt.
Add in the cooked chicken, onion, spinach, basil, and combine well.
Add the cheese and mix again.
Pour the mixture onto your muffin liners.
Bake for about 25 minutes.
Serve at room temperature.

Nutrition: Calories: 388; Fat: 25.8g; Carbs: 8.6g; Protein: 25.3g.

7. Green Pineapple

Preparation Time: 5 minutes

Cooking Time: 0 minutes

Servings: 3

Ingredients:

- ½ pineapple
- 1 broccoli, diced
- 1 cup water
- 1 long cucumber, diced
- A dash of salt
- 1 kiwi, diced

Directions:

Add kiwi, cucumber, pineapple, broccoli, and water in a blender.
Add the salt and blend until smooth.
Serve.

Nutrition: Calories: 251; Fat: 0.4g; Protein: 0.5g; Carbs: 22g.

8. Wholesome Mushroom and Cauliflower Risotto

Preparation Time: 15 minutes

Cooking Time: 7 minutes

Servings: 4

Ingredients:

- 1 medium cauliflower head, cut into florets
- 1 lb. shiitake mushrooms, sliced
- 3 medium garlic cloves, peeled and minced
- 2 tbsps. coconut aminos
- 1 cup homemade low-sodium chicken stock
- 1 cup full-fat coconut milk
- 1 tbsp. coconut oil, melted
- 1 small onion, finely chopped
- 2 tbsps. almond flour
- ¼ cup nutritional yeast

Directions:

On the Instant Pot, press "Sauté "and add the coconut oil.
Once hot, add the garlic, mushrooms, and onions. Sauté for 5 minutes or until softened, stirring occasionally.
Add the remaining ingredients except for the almond flour. Cover and cook for 2 minutes on high pressure.
When done, release the pressure naturally and remove the lid.
Sprinkle the almond flour over the risotto and stir to thicken. Serve and enjoy!

Nutrition: Calories: 230; Carbs: 8g; Protein: 7.5g; Fat: 18g.

9. Morning Meatloaf

Preparation Time: 10 minutes

Cooking Time: 25 minutes

Servings: 6

Ingredients:

- 1½ lbs. breakfast sausage
- 6 large organic eggs
- 2 tbsps. unsweetened non-dairy milk
- 1 small onion, finely chopped
- 2 medium garlic cloves, peeled and minced

- 4 oz. cream cheese, softened and cubed
- 1 cup shredded cheddar cheese
- 2 tbsps. scallions, chopped
- 1 cup water

Directions:

Add all the ingredients apart from water in a large bowl. Stir until well combined.

Form the sausage mixture into a meatloaf and wrap it with a sheet of aluminum foil. Ensure that the meatloaf fits inside your Instant Pot. If not, remove parts of the mixture and reserve them for future use.

Once you wrap the meatloaf into a packet, add 1 cup of water and a trivet to your Instant Pot. Put the meatloaf on the trivet's top.

Cover and cook for 25 minutes on high pressure. When done, quickly release the pressure. Carefully remove the lid.

Unwrap the meatloaf and check if the meatloaf is done. Serve and enjoy!

Nutrition: Calories: 592; Carbs: 2.5g; Protein: 11g; Fat: 49.5g.

10. Keto Oatmeal

Preparation Time: 10 minutes

Cooking Time: 3 minutes

Servings: 2

Ingredients:

- 1 cup unsweetened coconut milk
- 1 tbsp. coconut butter or ghee
- 1 tbsp. whole flax seeds

- 1 tbsp. chia seeds
- 1 tbsp. sunflower seeds
- ⅛ tsp. fine sea salt
- Blueberries (for garnish)

Directions:

Put all the ingredients into the Instant Pot and mix.

Cover and cook for 3 minutes on high pressure.

When done, quickly release the pressure and remove the lid.

Transfer to a bowl and top with blueberries. Serve and enjoy!

Nutrition: Calories: 353; Fat: 37.2g; Carbs: 4.1g; Protein: 3.7g.

11. Cinnamon and Pecan Porridge

Preparation Time: 10 minutes

Cooking Time: 9 minutes

Servings: 2

Ingredients:

- 1 cup unsweetened coconut milk
- ¼ cup almond butter
- 1 tbsp. coconut oil, melted
- 2 tbsps. whole chia seeds
- 2 tbsps. hemp seeds

- ¼ cup pecans, chopped
- ¼ cup walnuts, chopped
- ¼ cup unsweetened and toasted coconut
- 1 tsp. cinnamon

Directions:

Put all the ingredients into the Instant Pot and mix.

Cover and cook for 9 minutes on high pressure.

When done, release the pressure naturally and remove the lid. Serve and enjoy!

Nutrition: Calories: 580; Carbs: 11g; Protein: 32g; Fat: 51.7g.

12. Awesome Oatmeal

Preparation Time: 5 minutes

Cooking Time: 9 minutes

Servings: 4

Ingredients:

- 1 cup unsweetened coconut flakes
- 2 tbsps. butter or coconut oil
- ½ cup hemp seeds
- 2 tbsps. coconut flour
- 1 cup water

- ⅔ cups coconut cream
- ½ tbsp. ground cinnamon
- 1 tsp. pure vanilla extract
- 1 tbsp. pure pumpkin pureed
- 1 tsp. finely grated ginger
- A small pinch of sea salt

Directions:

Put all the ingredients into the Instant Pot and give a good stir.

Cover and cook for 9 minutes on high pressure. When done, allow for a full natural release. Carefully remove the lid.

Stir the oatmeal again and allow it to cool. Serve and enjoy!

Nutrition: Calories: 375; Carbs: 4g; Protein: 12g; Fat: 33g.

13. Grapefruit Yogurt Parfait

Preparation Time: 10 minutes

Cooking Time: 5 minutes

Servings: 4

Ingredients:

- ½ cup amaranth
- 1 grapefruit, peeled, separated into segments, deseeded, chopped
- 3 tbsps. toasted coconut
- Stevia to taste (optional)
- 1 cup plain, nonfat yogurt

Directions:

Place a pan over medium heat. Add amaranth and let it pop. It should take 3-5 minutes. Let it cool for a few minutes.

Add yogurt into a bowl. Add stevia and stir. Add 2 tablespoons of yogurt into each of 4 glasses. Place a layer of grapefruit in each glass. Add 1 tablespoon of popped amaranth and sprinkle some coconut into the glasses.

Repeat steps 2-3 until all the ingredients are used up.

Nutrition: Calories: 103g; Fat: 4g; Fiber: 1g; Carbs: 3g; Protein: 22g.

14. Creamy Mango and Banana Overnight Oats

Preparation Time: 10 minutes

Cooking Time: 0 minutes

Servings: 1

Ingredients:

For the Smoothie:

- 1 ripe banana
- ½ mango, peeled, cubed
- ½ tbsp. ground flaxseed
- 1 cup almond milk

For the Oats:

- ⅓ cup oats
- 1 small ripe banana, mashed
- ½ cup almond milk
- ½ tbsp. ground flaxseed
- 2 tbsps. chia seeds
- Stevia or erythritol to taste

Directions:

Add all the smoothie ingredients into a blender and blend until smooth.
Pour into a tall glass.
To make the oats layer: Add oats, almond milk, flaxseed, chia seeds and stevia into a bowl. Stir well and add banana. Mix until well combined. Pour it over the smoothie in the glass.
Chill in the refrigerator overnight and serve.

Nutrition: Calories: 199; Fat: 8g; Fiber: 4g; Carbs: 9g; Protein: 4g.

15. Bacon and Eggs with Tomatoes

Preparation Time: 10 minutes

Cooking Time: 20 minutes

Servings: 5

Ingredients:

- 4 large ripe tomatoes, halved
- 8 rashers smoked back bacon, defatted
- 4 eggs
- Salt to taste
- Pepper to taste
- 1 tsp. vinegar

Directions:

Set up the grill to preheat. Let it preheat to high heat.
Place a rack on the grill pan. Line the pan with foil. Place tomatoes on the rack. Let it grill for 3 minutes. Place bacon along with the tomatoes.
Grill for 4 minutes until soft.
Meanwhile, place a large saucepan over medium-high heat. Fill the saucepan up to about ¾ with water. Let it boil.
When it begins to boil, add vinegar and stir. Crack an egg into a bowl and slowly slide the egg into the boiling water. Repeat this, one at a time.
Cook each egg until it is soft boiled, for 2-3 minutes.
Meanwhile, divide the bacon and tomatoes into 2 plates.
Remove the eggs with a slotted spoon and place them on the plates. Sprinkle salt and pepper and serve.

Nutrition: Calories: 110; Fat: 10g; Fiber: 1g; Carbs: 3g; Protein: 6g.

16. Cinnamon Porridge

| **Preparation Time:** 10 minutes | **Cooking Time:** 30 minutes | **Servings:** 4 |

Ingredients:

- 4½ oz. jumbo porridge oats
- 20 oz. semi-skimmed milk
- 1 tsp. lemon juice
- ½ tsp. ground cinnamon + extra to garnish
- 2 ripe medium pears, peeled, cored, grated

Directions:

Add oats, milk and cinnamon into a nonstick saucepan. Place the saucepan over medium-low heat. Cook until creamy. Stir constantly.

Divide into bowls. Scatter pear on top. Drizzle lemon juice on top. Garnish with cinnamon and serve.

Nutrition: Calories: 383; Fat: 14g; Fiber: 4g; Carbs: 3g; Protein: 8g.

---

17. Sesame-Seared Salmon

| **Preparation Time:** 5 minutes | **Cooking Time:** 7 minutes | **Servings:** 4 |

Ingredients:

- 4 wild salmon fillets (about 1lb.)
- 1½ tbsps. Sesame seeds
- 2 tbsps. Toasted sesame oil
- 1½ tbsps. Avocado oil
- 1 tsp. sea salt

Directions:

Using a paper towel or a clean kitchen towel, pat the fillets to dry. Brush each with 1 tablespoon of sesame oil and season with a half teaspoon of salt.

Place a large skillet over medium-high heat and drizzle with avocado oil. Once the oil is hot, add the salmon fillets with the flesh side down. Cook for about 3 minutes and flip. Cook the skin side for an additional 3-4 minutes, without overcooking it.

Remove the pan from the heat and brush with the remaining sesame oil. Season with the remaining salt and sprinkle with sesame seeds. Best served with a green salad.

Nutrition: Calories: 291; Fat: 14g; Fiber: 6g; Carbs: 3g; Protein: 8g.

---

18. Eggs and Salsa

Preparation Time: 5 minutes

Cooking Time: 5 minutes

Servings: 2

Ingredients:

- 3 cups tomatoes
- 1 green onion (bunch)
- 1 bunch cilantro, chopped
- 1 cup red onion, chopped
- 1 lime

- 2 small habanero chilies, chopped
- 2 garlic cloves, minced
- 8 eggs, whisked
- 1 tsp. olive oil
- Sea salt to taste

Directions:

Mix tomatoes, green onions, red onion, habaneros, garlic, cilantro, lime juice and toss well.
Add a pinch of salt, toss again and keep this in the fridge until you serve it.
Heat up a pan with a drizzle of oil, add eggs, and scramble them for 4-5 minutes.
Divide scrambled eggs among plates, add salsa on top and serve.

Nutrition: Calories: 383; Fat: 14g; Fiber: 4g; Carbs: 3g; Protein: 8g.

19. Poached Egg

Preparation Time: 5 minutes

Cooking Time: 5 minutes

Servings: 3

Ingredients:

- 1 tbsp. rice vinegar
- 1 egg

- Salt to taste
- Black pepper to taste

Directions:

Put some water into a pot and heat up.
Simmer gently, add vinegar, and whisk.
Crack the egg into simmering water and cook for 5 minutes making sure it stays in a compact shape.
Transfer egg to a plate and serve for breakfast.

Nutrition: Calories: 200; Fat: 8g; Fiber: 2g; Carbs: 8g; Protein: 6g.

20. Cheesy Egg Muffins

Preparation Time: 20 minutes.

Cooking Time: 10

minutes.   **Servings:** 6

Ingredients:
- 4 eggs, large
- 2 tablespoons Greek-yogurt, full fat
- 3 tablespoons almond flour
- 1/4 teaspoon baking powder
- 1and 1/2 cup cheddar cheese, shredded

Directions:
1. Set your oven to preheat to 375°F. Add yogurt and eggs to a medium bowl, season with salt, pepper, then whisk to combine.
2. Add baking powder and coconut flour, then mix to form a smooth batter. Finally, add your cheese, and fold to combine.
3. Pour your mixture evenly into 6 silicone muffin cups and set to bake in your preheated oven.
4. Allow baking until your eggs are fully set and lightly golden on top, about 20 minutes, turning the tray at the halfway point.
5. Allow muffins to cool on a cooling rack, then serve. Enjoy.

Nutrition: Calories: 144; Carbs: 1.43g ;Protein: 8g;Fats: 11.9g

CHAPTER 11: LUNCH

21. Salmon with Sauce

Preparation Time: 5 minutes   **Cooking Time:** 15 minutes   **Servings:** 2

Ingredients:

- 1½ lb. salmon fillet
- 1 tbsp. duck fat
- ¾ to 1 tsp. dried dill weed
- ¾ to 1 tsp. dried tarragon
- ¼ cup Heavy cream
- 2 tbsps. butter
- Salt and pepper to taste

Directions:

Slice the salmon in half and make 2 fillets. Season skin side with salt and pepper and meat of the fish with spices.

In a skillet, heat 1 tbsp. duck fat over medium heat.

Add salmon to the hot pan, skin side down.

Cook the salmon for about 5 minutes. When the skin is crisp, lower the heat and flip the salmon.

Cook salmon on low heat for 7 to 15 minutes or until your desired doneness is reached.

Remove salmon from the pan and set aside.

Add spices and butter to the pan and let brown. Once browned, add cream and mix.

Top salmon with sauce and serve.

Nutrition: Calories: 449; Total Fat: 34.5g; Saturated Fat: 14.4g; Cholesterol: 136mg; Sodium: 168mg; Total Carbs: 1.1g; Dietary Fiber: 0.1g; Total Sugars: 0g; Protein: 35.2g.

22. Butter Chicken

Preparation Time: 5 minutes   **Cooking Time:** 24 minutes   **Servings:** 4

Ingredients:

- ¼ cup butter
- 2 cups mushrooms, sliced
- 4 large chicken thighs
- ½ tsp. onion powder
- ½ tsp. garlic powder
- 1 tsp. kosher salt
- ¼ tsp black pepper
- ½ cup water
- 1 tsp. Dijon mustard
- 1 tbsp. fresh tarragon, chopped

Directions:

Season the chicken thighs with onion powder, garlic powder, salt, and pepper.

In a sauté pan, melt 1 tbsp. of butter.

Sear the chicken thighs for about 3 to 4 minutes per side, or until both sides are golden brown.

Remove the thighs from the pan.

Add the remaining 2 tbsps. of butter to the pan and melt.

Add the mushrooms and cook for 4 to 5 minutes or until golden brown. Stirring as little as possible.

Add the Dijon mustard and water to the pan. Stir to deglaze.

Place the chicken thighs back in the pan with the skin side up.

Cover and simmer for 15 minutes.

Stir in the fresh herbs. Let sit for 5 minutes and serve.

Nutrition: Calories: 414; Total Fat: 32.9g; Saturated Fat: 13.6g; Cholesterol: 149mg; Sodium: 786mg; Total Carbs: 2g; Dietary Fiber: 0.5g; Total Sugars: 0.8g; Protein: 26.5g.

23. Lamb Curry

Preparation Time: 10 minutes

Cooking Time: 4 hours

Servings: 6

Ingredients:

- 2 tbsps. fresh ginger, grated
- 2 garlic cloves, peeled and minced
- 2 tsps. cardamom
- 1 onion peeled and chopped
- 6 cloves
- 1 lb. lamb meat, cubed
- 2 tsps. cumin powder
- 1 tsp. garam masala
- ½ tsp. chili powder
- 1 tsp. turmeric
- 2 tsps. coriander
- 1 lb. spinach
- 14 oz. canned tomatoes

Directions:

In a slow cooker, mix lamb with tomatoes, spinach, ginger, garlic, onion, cardamom, cloves, cumin, garam masala, chili, turmeric, and coriander.

Stir well. Cover and cook on high for 4 hours.

Uncover the slow cooker, stir the chili, divide into bowls, and serve.

Nutrition: Calories: 186; Total Fat: 7.2g; Saturated Fat: 2.5g; Cholesterol: 38mg; Sodium: 477mg; Total Carbs: 16.3g; Dietary Fiber: 5g; Total Sugars: 5g; Protein: 14.4g.

24. Zuppa Toscana with Cauliflower

Preparation Time: 5 minutes

Cooking Time: 25 minutes

Servings: 4

Ingredients:

- 1 lb. ground Italian sausage
- 6 cups homemade low-sodium chicken stock
- 2 cups cauliflower florets
- 1 onion, finely chopped
- 1 cup kale, stemmed and roughly chopped

- 1 (14.5 oz.) can full-fat coconut milk
- ¼ tsp. sea salt
- ¼ tsp. freshly cracked black pepper

Directions:

On the Instant Pot, press "Sauté" and add the ground Italian sausage. Cook until brown, stirring occasionally and breaking up the meat with a wooden spoon.

Add the remaining ingredients except for the kale and coconut milk and stir until well combined. Cover and cook for 10 minutes on high pressure. When done, release the pressure naturally and remove the lid. Stir in the kale and coconut milk. Cover and sit for 5 minutes or until the kale has wilted. Serve and enjoy!

Nutrition: Calories: 653; Carbs: 8g; Protein: 26g; Fat: 4g.

25. Pork Carnitas

Preparation Time: 20 minutes

Cooking Time: 1 hour and 24 minutes

Servings: 4

Ingredients:

- 6 medium garlic cloves, minced
- 2 tsps. ground cumin
- 1 tsp. smoked paprika
- 3 chipotle peppers in adobo sauce, minced
- 1 tsp. dried oregano
- 2 bay leaves

- 1 cup homemade low-sodium chicken broth
- Fine sea salt and freshly cracked black pepper
- 2 tbsps. olive oil
- 2½ lbs. boneless pork shoulder, cut into 4 large pieces

Directions:

Season the pork shoulder with sea salt, black pepper, ground cumin, dried oregano, and smoked paprika.

On the Instant Pot, press "Sauté" and add the olive oil.

Once hot, add the pork pieces and sear for 4 minutes per side or until brown.

Add the remaining ingredients inside your Instant Pot. Cover and cook for 80 minutes on high pressure. When done, quickly release the pressure and remove the lid.

Carefully shred the pork using 2 forks and continue to stir until well coated with the liquid.

Remove the bay leave and adjust the seasoning if necessary. Serve and enjoy!

Nutrition: Calories: 170; Carbs: 2g; Protein: 4g; Fat: 8g.

26. Cheesy Taco Skillet

Preparation Time: 10 minutes

Cooking Time: 20 minutes

Servings: 4

Ingredients:

- 1 lb. lean grass-fed ground beef
- 1 large yellow or white onion, finely chopped
- 2 medium-sized bell peppers, finely chopped
- 1 (12 oz.) can have diced tomatoes with green chilies

- 2 large zucchinis, finely chopped
- 2 tbsps. taco seasoning
- 3 cups fresh baby kale or fresh spinach
- 1½ cups shredded cheddar cheese or shredded jack cheese

Directions:

In a large nonstick skillet, add the ground beef and cook until lightly brown. Drain the excess grease.

Add the chopped onions, chopped bell peppers, diced tomatoes with green chilies, zucchini, and taco seasoning. Cook for 5 minutes, stirring occasionally.

Add the fresh baby kale or spinach. Cook until wilted.

Cover with 1½ cups of shredded cheddar cheese and cover with a lid.

Once the cheese has melted, serve and enjoy!

Nutrition: Calories: 287; Fat: 8g; Fiber: 2g; Carbs: 12g; Protein: 28g.

27. Mini Thai Lamb Salad Bites

Preparation Time: 10 minutes

Cooking Time: 8 minutes

Servings: 15

Ingredients:

- 1 large cucumber, cut into 0.39-inch-thick diagonal rounds

- ½ lb. (250 g.) lamb blackstrap

- ¾ cup cherry tomatoes quartered
- ⅓ cup fresh mint, loosely packed
- ⅓ cup fresh coriander, loosely packed
- ¼ small red onion, finely diced
- 1 tsp. fish sauce
- Juice 1 lime
- Coconut oil

Directions:

Place pan over medium heat and heat oil. Cook the lamb for 4 minutes on each side. Remove from heat and let it rest.

In a mixing bowl, toss the onions, tomatoes, mint, coriander, fish sauce, and lime juice.

Cut the lamb into thin strips and add to the salad bowl. Toss to combine.

Spoon the mixture on each cucumber cut. Chill and serve.

Nutrition: Calories: 58; Fat: 2g; Fiber: 2g; Carbs: 20g; Protein: 5g.

28. Bacon Egg and Sausage Cups

Preparation Time: 10 minutes

Cooking Time: 20 minutes

Servings: 8

Ingredients:

- 3 oz. breakfast sausages
- 2 slices bacon, chopped
- 4 large eggs
- 2 large green onions, chopped
- 1 oz. cheddar cheese, shredded
- 1 tbsp. coconut oil

Directions:

Preheat oven to 350°F.

Grease your muffin pan and set it aside.

In a mixing bowl, beat the eggs together with the cheese. Set aside.

Brown the bacon in a nonstick skillet over medium heat. Add the crumbled sausage and cook until no longer pink.

Add the onion and cook until wilted. Remove the skillet from the heat and let it cool for 1–2 minutes.

Add the meat mixture to the egg mixture and beat well using a spoon.

Scoop mixture into the greased muffin pan and bake for 15–20 minutes or until the tops begin to brown. Remove from pan and serve.

Nutrition: Calories: 100; Fat: 8g; Fiber: 2g; Carbs: 20g; Protein: 5g.

29. Smoked Salmon and Avocado Stacks

Preparation Time: 15 minutes

Cooking Time: 0 minutes

Servings: 6

Ingredients:

- ½ lb. smoked salmon, finely diced
- 1 ripe avocado, seed removed and diced

- 1 tbsp. chives, chopped
- Fresh or dried dill leaves
- 3 tsps. fresh lemon juice
- Black pepper, cracked

Directions:

Combine salmon, chives, and 1 tsp. of lemon juice in a small mixing bowl.

In another mixing bowl, toss the avocado, remaining lemon juice, and pepper.

Using a presentation ring, arrange the stacks on the serving plates. Arrange the avocado at the bottom and top it with the salmon mixture and gently press. Remove the mold and garnish the stack with dill leaves. Serve chilled.

Nutrition: Calories: 106; Fat: 12g; Fiber: 2g; Carbs: 20g; Protein: 5g.

30. Homemade Turkey Burger and Relish

Preparation Time: 10 minutes

Cooking Time: 15 minutes

Servings: 4

Ingredients:

- 2 lbs. ground turkey, made into 4 patties
- 1 onion, finely chopped
- 1 red bell pepper, chopped up finely

- 3 cups red cabbage, chopped or shredded
- 1 tbsp. olive oil
- ¼ cup balsamic vinegar
- ¼ tsp. garlic salt
- 4 lettuce leaves, large if possible

Directions:

Take a large skillet pan and place over medium heat.

Add the olive oil and allow it to reach temperature.

Add the onion, red cabbage, and pepper to the pan and cook until everything until softened.

Now add the balsamic vinegar and the garlic salt and combine everything, letting it simmer for a few minutes until the contents have been caramelized from the vinegar.

Remove the contents of the pan and set them aside to cool.

Take your turkey patties and season with salt and pepper.

Cook your patties for around 4 minutes on each side in either a pan or under the grill.

Once cooked, transfer each patty onto a lettuce leaf and add some of the relishes on top.

Nutrition: Calories: 442; Protein: 47.86g; Fat: 21.17g; Carbs: 16.93g.

31. Butternut Squash Risotto

Preparation Time: 10 minutes

Cooking Time: 15 minutes

Servings: 4

Ingredients:

- 2 tbsps. butter
- 2 tbsps. minced sage
- ¼ tsp. black pepper, ground
- 1 tsp. minced rosemary
- 1 tsp. salt
- ½ cup dry sherry
- 4 cups riced cauliflower
- ½ cup butternut squash, cooked and mashed
- ½ cup Parmesan cheese, grated
- ½ cup Mascarpone cheese
- ⅛ tsp. grated nutmeg
- 1 tsp. minced garlic

Directions:

Melt your butter inside of a large frying pan turned to a medium level of heat.

Add your rosemary, your sage, and garlic. Cook this for about 1 minute or until this mixture begins to become fragrant.

Add in the cauliflower rice, pepper, salt, and mashed squash. Cook this for 3 minutes. You will know it is ready for the next step when cauliflower starts to soften up for you.

Add in your sherry and cook this for an additional 6 minutes, or until the majority of the liquid is absorbed into the rice, or when the cauliflower is much softer.

Stir in the Mascarpone cheese, Parmesan cheese, as well as nutmeg (grated).

Cook all of this on a medium heat level, being sure to stir it occasionally and do this until the cheese has melted and the risotto has gotten creamy. That will take around 4–5 minutes.

Taste the risotto and add more pepper and salt to season if you wish.

Remove your pan from the burner and garnish your risotto with more of the herbs as well as some grated parmesan.

Serve and enjoy

Nutrition: Calories: 337; Fat: 25g; Carbs: 9g; Protein: 8g.

32. Chicken in Sweet and Sour Sauce with Corn Salad

Preparation Time: 10 minutes

Cooking Time: 23 minutes

Servings: 4

Ingredients:

- 2 cups plus 2 tbsps. unflavored low-fat yogurt
- 2 cups frozen mango chunks
- 3 tbsps. honey
- ¼ cup plus 1 tbsp. apple cider vinegar
- ¼ cup sultana
- 2 tbsps. olive oil, plus an amount to be brushed
- ¼ tsp. cayenne pepper
- 5 dried tomatoes (not in oil)
- 2 small cloves garlic, finely chopped
- 4 cobs, peeled
- 8 peeled and boned chicken legs, peeled (about 700g)
- 6 cups mixed salad
- 2 medium carrots, finely sliced

Directions:

For the smoothie: in a blender, mix 2 cups of yogurt, 2 cups of ice, 1 cup of mango, and all the honey until the mixture becomes completely smooth. Divide into 4 glasses and refrigerate until ready to use. Rinse the blender.

Preheat the grill to medium-high heat. Mix the remaining cup of mango, ¼ cup water, ¼ cup vinegar, sultanas, olive oil, cayenne pepper, tomatoes, and garlic in a microwave bowl. Cover with a piece of clear film and cook in the microwave until the tomatoes become soft, for about 3 minutes. Leave to cool slightly and pass in a blender. Transfer to a small bowl. Leave 2 tablespoons aside to garnish, turn the chicken into the remaining mixture.

Put the corn on the grill, cover, and bake, turning it over if necessary, until it is burnt, about 10 minutes. Remove and keep warm.

Brush the grill over medium heat and brush the grills with a little oil. Turn the chicken legs into half the remaining sauce and ½ teaspoon of salt. Put on the grill and cook until the cooking marks appear and the internal temperature reaches 75°C on an instantaneous thermometer, 8 to 10 minutes per side. Bart and sprinkle a few times with the remaining sauce while cooking.

While the chicken is cooking, beat the remaining 2 tablespoons of yogurt, the 2 tablespoons of sauce set aside, the remaining spoonful of vinegar, 1 tablespoon of water, and ¼ teaspoon of salt in a large bowl. Mix the mixed salad with the carrots. Divide chicken, corn, and salad into 4 serving dishes. Garnish the salad with the dressing set aside. Serve each plate with a mango smoothie.

Nutrition: Calories: 346; Protein: 56g; Fat: 45g.

33. Asparagus and Pistachios Vinaigrette

Preparation Time: 10 minutes

Cooking Time: 15 minutes

Servings: 2

Ingredients:

- 2 bunches (455g) large asparagus, without the tip
- 1 tbsp. olive oil
- Salt and freshly ground black pepper
- 6 tbsps. sliced pistachios blanched and boiled
- 1½ tbsps. lemon juice
- ¼ tsp. sugar
- 1½ tsps. lemon zest

Directions:

Preheat the oven to 220°C. Put the grill in the top third of the oven. Place the asparagus on a baking tray covered with baking paper. Sprinkle with olive oil and season with a little salt and pepper. Bake for 15 minutes, until soft.

Meanwhile, blend 5 tablespoons of almonds, lemon juice, sugar, and 6 tablespoons of water for 1 minute until smooth. Taste and regulate salt. Pour the sauce on a plate and put the spinach on the sauce. Decorate with peel and the remaining spoon of pistachios

Nutrition: Calories: 560; Fat: 5g; Fiber: 2g; Carbs: 3g; Protein: 9g.

34. Chinese Chicken Salad

Preparation Time: 15 minutes

Cooking Time: 45 minutes

Servings: 4

Ingredients:

For the Chicken Salad:

- 4 divided chicken breasts with skin and bones
- 1 tbsp. olive oil
- Salt and freshly ground black pepper
- 500g asparagus, with the ends removed and cut into 3 parts diagonally
- 1 red pepper, peeled
- Chinese condiment, recipe to follow
- 2 spring onions (both the white and the green part), sliced diagonally
- 1 tbsp. white sesame seeds, toasted

For Chinese Dressing:

- 120 ml vegetable oil
- 60 ml apple cider vinegar
- 60 ml soy sauce
- 1½ tbsp. black sesame
- ½ tbsp. honey
- 1 clove garlic, minced
- ½ tsp. fresh peeled and grated ginger
- ½ tbsp. sesame seeds, toasted
- 60g peanut butter
- 2 tsps. salt
- ½ tsp. freshly ground black pepper

Directions:

For the chicken salad: Heat the oven to 180°C (or 200°C for a gas oven). Put the chicken breast on a baking tray and rub the skin with a little olive oil. Season freely with salt and pepper.

Brown for 35 to 40 minutes, until the chicken is freshly cooked. Let it cool down as long as it takes to handle it. Remove the meat from the bones, remove the skin and chop the chicken into medium-sized pieces.

Blanch the asparagus in a pot of salted water for 3-5 minutes until tender. Soak them in water with ice to stop cooking. Drain them. Cut the peppers into strips the same size as the asparagus. In a large bowl, mix the chopped chicken, asparagus and peppers.

Spread the Chinese dressing on chicken and vegetables. Add the spring onions and sesame seeds, and season to taste. Serve cold or at room temperature.

For Chinese dressing: Mix all ingredients and set aside until use.

Nutrition: Calories: 222; Protein: 2g; Fat: 10g; Sugar 6g.

35. Garlic Butter Beef Steak

Preparation Time: 5 minutes

Cooking Time: 15 minutes

Servings: 2

Ingredients:

- 1 lb. beef sirloin steaks
- ½ cup red wine
- 4 tbsps. unsalted butter
- 2 tbsps. fresh parsley, finely chopped
- 4 medium garlic cloves, peeled and minced
- Fine sea salt and freshly cracked black pepper

Directions:

Season the beef steaks with sea salt and freshly cracked black pepper.

On the Instant Pot, press "Sauté" and add the butter. Once melted, add the beef steaks and sear for 2 minutes per side or until brown.

Pour in the red wine and fresh parsley. Cover and cook for 12 minutes on high pressure. When done, release the pressure naturally and carefully remove the lid.

Top the steak with butter sauce. Serve and enjoy!

Nutrition: Calories: 337; Carbs: 2.5g; Protein: 34.5g; Fat: 18.7g.

36. Instant Pot Teriyaki Chicken

Cooking Time: 25 minutes

Preparation Time: 5 minutes

Servings: 4

Ingredients:

- ½ cup soy sauce
- ½ cup water
- ½ cup brown sugar
- 2 tbsps. rice wine vinegar
- 1 tbsp. mirin (Japanese sweet wine)
- 1 tbsp. sake
- 1 tbsp. minced garlic

- 1 dash freshly cracked black pepper
- 1 lb. skinless, boneless chicken

Directions:

Combine soy sauce, brown sugar, water, rice wine vinegar, sake, mirin, pepper, and garlic in a bowl to prepare the sauce.

Put chicken in an electric pressure cooker (such as Instant Pot(R)). Pour the sauce over.

Close lid and lock. Set to Meat function, with the timer on to 12 minutes. Give 10-15 minutes for pressure to build.

Gently release pressure with the quick-release method according to the manufacturer's instructions, for 5 minutes. Remove lid. Insert the instant-read thermometer into the middle of the chicken and make sure to reach at least 165°F (74°C). If not hot enough, cook for 2-4 more minutes.

Take chicken out from the cooker. Shred or cut up. Mix with sauce from the pot.

Nutrition: Calories: 259; Carbs: 33.1g; Protein: 24.3g; Fat: 2.3g.

37. Teriyaki Salmon

Preparation Time: 15 minutes   **Cooking Time:** 8 minutes   **Servings:** 2

Ingredients:

- 3 tbsps. lime juice
- 2 tbsps. olive oil
- 2 tbsps. reduced-sodium teriyaki sauce
- 1 tbsp. balsamic vinegar
- 1 tbsp. Dijon mustard
- 1 tsp. garlic powder
- 6 drops hot pepper sauce
- 6 uncooked jumbo salmon

Directions:

Mix together all ingredients except the salmon in a big ziplock plastic bag then put in the shrimp. Seal the zip lock bag and turn to coat the salmon. Keep in the fridge for an hour and occasionally turn.

Drain the marinated salmon and discard the marinade. Broil the salmon 4 inches from heat for 3 to 4 minutes per side or until the salmon turn pink in color.

Nutrition: Calories: 93; Carbs: 3g; Protein: 13g; Fat: 4g.

38. Creamy Lamb Korma

Preparation Time: 5 minutes   **Cooking Time:** 16 minutes   **Servings:** 4

Ingredients:

- 1 lb. lamb steak, cut into 1-inch pieces
- 1 tbsp. extra-virgin olive oil
- 1 medium onion, finely chopped
- 1-inch piece ginger, peeled and minced
- 6 medium garlic cloves, peeled and minced
- 2 tbsps. tomato paste
- ½ cup coconut milk or plain yogurt
- ¾ cups water
- 3 tsps. garam masala
- ½ tsp. turmeric powder
- 1 tsp. smoked or regular paprika
- ½ tsp. cardamom powder
- ¼ tsp. sea salt
- ¼ tsp. freshly cracked black pepper

Directions:

On the Instant Pot, press "Sauté" and add the olive oil. Once hot, add the chopped onions, minced garlic, and minced ginger. Sauté for 1 minute, stirring frequently.
Add the tomato paste along with ¼ cup of water. Give a good stir.
Stir in all the seasonings and give another good stir.
Stir in the coconut milk, the remainder of the water, and the lamb pieces. Cover and cook for 15 minutes on high pressure. When done, release the pressure naturally and remove the lid.
Serve and enjoy!

Nutrition: Calories: 280; Carbs: 5g; Protein: 26g; Fat: 25g.

39. Simple Roasted Cabbage

Preparation Time: 4 minutes   **Cooking Time:** 25 minutes   **Servings:** 4

Ingredients:

- 1 green cabbage head, shredded and cut into large wedges
- 2 tablespoons olive oil
- 1 tablespoon cilantro, chopped
- 1 tablespoon lemon juice
- A pinch of salt and black pepper

Directions:

1. Preheat your air fryer at 370 degrees F, add the cabbage wedges mixed with all the ingredients in the basket and cook for 25 minutes.
2. Divide between plates and serve as a side dish.

Nutrition: 185 Calorie; 6g Fat; 3g Fiber; 4g Protein

CHAPTER 12: DINNER

40. Maple Walnut-Glazed Black-Eyed Peas with Collard Greens

Preparation Time: 10 minutes | **Cooking Time:** 15 minutes | **Servings:** 3

Ingredients:

For the Maple-Walnut Glaze:

- ¾ cup water
- ½ cup walnuts, chopped
- ½ tbsp. Tamari sauce
- 2 tbsps. sugar-free maple syrup
- 1 tsp. arrowroot starch flour
- 1 tsp. nutmeg
- ½ tsp. ground mustard
- ⅛ tsp. ground ginger
- ⅛ tsp. ground cinnamon
- ⅛ tsp. ground cloves

For the Black-Eyed Peas and Collard Greens:

- 4 cups cooked black-eyed peas
- 1 large bunch fresh collard greens, cleaned, stems removed, and chopped
- ¼ cup water (plus more)

Directions:

For the maple-walnut glaze, put all ingredients in a blender in this order: water, walnuts, tamari, maple syrup, starch, and spices. Blend starting at the lowest setting and gradually adjust to the highest. Blend on high for about 40 seconds. Set aside.

For the peas and collards, place a 5-quart sauté pan over medium-high heat and add water. Put the collards and steam-sauté until tender, about 10 minutes. You can also adjust the doneness according to your preference.

Add the glaze to the greens and continue to cook on medium-high for about 2 minutes. Stir frequently.

Add the peas. Continue to cook and stir for another minute. Serve immediately.

Nutrition: Calories: 233; Fat: 8g; Fiber: 2g; Carbs: 8g; Protein: 13g.

41. Filipino Chicken Adobo

Preparation Time: 10 minutes | **Cooking Time:** 15 minutes | **Servings:** 4

Ingredients:

- 1 lb. boneless chicken, cut into pieces
- 2 tbsps. soy sauce
- 3 tbsps. apple cider vinegar
- 1½ tsps. garlic, minced
- 2 tbsps. olive oil

Directions:

Mix the soy sauce, vinegar, garlic, and oil in a pan.

Add the chicken and coat it with the soy sauce mixture.

Place the pan over medium heat, add the chicken, cover with a lid, and let it simmer for 10-15 minutes.

Uncover the pan and adjust the heat to medium-high. Cook until the chicken is browned. Stir occasionally to avoid burning.

Serve and enjoy!

Nutrition: Calories: 207; Fat: 8g; Fiber: 2g; Carbs: 8g; Protein: 6g.

42. Kale & Artichoke Soup

Preparation Time: 10 minutes

Cooking Time: 30 minutes

Servings: 3

Ingredients:

- 2 cups artichoke hearts
- 2 cups kale leaves, tightly packed and stem discarded
- 32 oz. low sodium chicken broth
- ½ white sweet potato, chopped into ½-inch slices
- 1 cup unsweetened almond milk
- 1 large yellow onion, chopped
- 1 pinch cayenne pepper
- 1 pinch ground nutmeg
- 2 tbsps. Olive oil
- Sea salt

Directions:

Place a pot over medium heat and heat the oil. Sauté the onions for about 8-10 minutes or until translucent.

Put in the sweet potatoes and continue to cook, stirring frequently, until soft.

Add the artichoke hearts, broth, nutmeg, and cayenne. Season with salt and bring to a boil.

Lower the heat and simmer for 10 minutes.

Add the kale and cover the pot with a lid. Leave it for 1 minute until the kale leaves have wilted.

Add the almond milk. Next, using an immersion blender, process the mixture until smooth. Alternatively, transfer the soup to the blender and process in batches.

Strain the soup to separate the strands of artichoke hearts. Serve the soup hot or cold.

Drizzle with oil before serving.

Nutrition: Calories: 108; Fat: 8g; Fiber: 2g; Carbs: 8g; Protein: 7g.

43. Poached Eggs and Bacon on Toast

Preparation Time: 10 minutes

Cooking Time: 20 minutes

Servings: 1

Ingredients:

- 2 slices bacon
- 2 medium eggs
- Salmon (If you want)
- 200g baby spinach leaves
- Black pepper
- Sea salt
- 1 slice toast

Directions:

Make a large pan of water to a gentle boil.

Stir the water gently and then break the eggs; poach for 4 minutes or until the whites are set.

During that time, heat a deep frying pan, add a splash of water, and sprinkle with the spinach.

Cook for 2 minutes until the mixture is withered.

Take spinach and place it aside on a plate. Fry the bacon till golden brown.

Put the spinach and salmon on a toast, sprinkle with salt and pepper.

Cover all of it with poached eggs and bacon.

Nutrition: Calories: 270; Fat: 8g; Fiber: 2g; Carbs: 8g; Protein: 37g.

44. Asparagus and Green Peas Salad

Preparation Time: 10 minutes

Cooking Time: 30 minutes

Servings: 2

Ingredients:

- 1 cup green peas
- 1 carrot, chopped
- 1 lb. asparagus trimmed
- 1 bunch fries
- 1 red onion, chopped
- 1 rib celery, chopped
- 1 tbsp. flaxseed oil
- ½ tbsp. Dijon mustard
- 2 tbsps. balsamic vinegar
- 1 tbsp. extra-virgin olive oil
- ½ cup goat cheese, crumbled

Directions:

Preheat the oven to 450°F.

Pour 3 cups of water into a large saucepan and bring to a boil. Add in onion lentils, carrots, and celery. Reduce heat and allow to simmer for 15 minutes or until the lentils are tender. Drain. Set aside.

Meanwhile, layer asparagus on a baking sheet. Tilt sheet to roll asparagus to coat with cooking spray. Roast for 15 minutes.

In another bowl, put together mustard and balsamic vinegar. Whisk in flaxseed oil and olive oil. Mix well. Drizzle in lentil mixture. Toss until well coated.

To serve, arrange fries on plates. Put a lentil mixture and sprinkle goat cheese.

Nutrition: Calories: 156; Fat: 8g; Fiber: 2g; Carbs: 8g; Protein: 56g.

45. Quick and Easy Squash Soup

Preparation Time: 5 minutes

Cooking Time: 15 minutes

Servings: 1

Ingredients:

- 1 tbsp. olive oil
- 1 cup chopped onions
- 1 cup chopped squash
- 2 cups chicken broth
- ½ tsp. nutmeg
- ½ tsp. salt
- 1 tsp. pepper

Directions:

Deposit your 1 tablespoon of olive oil into a large saucepan, before adding your 1 cup of chopped onions, your 1 cup of chopped squash, your 2 cups of chicken broth, your ½ teaspoon of nutmeg, your ¼ teaspoon of salt, and your 1 teaspoon of pepper.

Stir everything together well and cook for 15 minutes under high heat.

Serve when ready!

Nutrition: Calories: 108; Fat: 8g; Fiber: 2g; Carbs: 8g; Protein: 7g.

46. Sesame-Ginger Chicken Salad

Preparation Time: 10 minutes

Cooking Time: 0 minutes

Servings: 2

Ingredients:

- 3 oz. cooked chicken breast, shredded
- 4 cups romaine lettuce, chopped
- ¼ cup carrot, shredded
- ½ cup fresh spinach
- ¼ cup radishes, sliced
- 1 scallion, sliced
- 3 tbsps. Sugar-free sesame-ginger dressing

Directions:

In a medium-sized salad bowl, mix all the ingredients (except for the sesame-ginger dressing) and toss well.
Add the dressing and toss well. Serve and enjoy!

Nutrition: Calories: 340; Fat: 8g; Fiber: 2g; Carbs: 8g; Protein: 6g.

47. Reds Salad on Bacon and Balsamic Vinaigrette

Preparation Time: 10 minutes

Cooking Time: 10 minutes

Servings: 3

Ingredients:

- 1 head red leaf lettuce, torn
- 2 red oak leaf lettuce, torn
- ½ cup radicchio, julienned
- 6 streaky bacon
- 2 tbsps. extra virgin olive oil
- ⅛ cup balsamic vinegar
- 2 garlic cloves, grated
- 1 tbsp. Dijon mustard
- A dash of red pepper flakes
- A pinch of sea salt, add more if needed
- A pinch of black pepper, add more if needed

Directions:

For the dressing, pour olive oil into a non-stick skillet. Fry streaky bacon for 3 minutes or until golden brown. Transfer to a plate and crumble into small pieces. Set aside
In the same pan, add garlic, balsamic vinegar, Dijon mustard, red pepper flakes, salt, and pepper. Whisk until mixture is well blended. Set aside
To assemble, in a big salad bowl, put together red leaf lettuce, red oak leaf lettuce, and radicchio. Drizzle in dressing. Top with bacon bits. Serve.

Nutrition: Calories: 108; Fat: 50g; Fiber: 2g; Carbs: 8g; Protein: 48g.

48. Veggie-Stuffed Omelet

Preparation Time: 10 minutes

Cooking Time: 15 minutes

Servings: 1

Ingredients:

- 2 eggs, beaten
- ¼ cup mushrooms, sliced
- 1 cup loosely packed contemporary baby spinach leaves, rinsed

- 2 tbsps. red bell pepper, chopped
- 1 tbsp. onion, chopped
- 1 tbsp. reduced-fat cheddar cheese, shredded
- 1 tsp. olive or canola oil
- 1 tbsp. water
- A dash of salt
- A dash of pepper

Directions:

Heat oil in an 8-inch non-stick skillet. Sauté the mushrooms, onion, and bell pepper for about 2 minutes until the onion is tender. Add the spinach and continue to cook, stirring frequently, until the spinach wilts. Once cooked, transfer the vegetables to a small bowl.

In a medium bowl, whisk the beaten eggs, water, salt, and pepper until well combined.

Place the same skillet in which you cooked the vegetable mixture over medium-high heat. Add the egg mixture immediately. Make a quick, sliding back-and-forth motion with the pan, using a spatula to spread the eggs at the bottom of the pan. Once the mixture is spread, let it stand for a few seconds to lightly brown the bottom of the omelet. Do not overcook it.

Carefully place the vegetable mixture on the half side of the omelet. Top it with cheese and, using a spatula, gently fold the other half over the vegetables. Transfer the veggie-stuffed omelet to a plate and serve.

Nutrition: Calories: 150; Fat: 8g; Fiber: 2g; Carbs: 8g; Protein: 24g.

49. Roasted Carrots and Cashew Salad on Lemon Vinaigrette

Preparation Time: 10 minutes

Cooking Time: 30 minutes

Servings: 2

Ingredients:

- 2 carrots, cubed
- ½ cup cashew nuts halved
- 2 tsps. cumin powder
- A pinch of sea salt
- A pinch of black pepper, to taste
- ½ tbsp. olive oil
- 1 tsp. extra virgin olive oil
- 1 lemon, juiced
- 1 tbsp. stevia
- 2 bags arugula, chopped
- 2 bags baby spinach, chopped

Directions:

Preheat the oven to 400°F. Line a baking sheet with parchment paper.

Put together olive oil, carrots, cumin powder, and cashew nuts in a bowl. Season with salt and pepper.

Place mixture onto the baking sheet. Roast for 30 minutes.

Remove from the kitchen appliance and permit to chill for a number of minutes.

To make the lemon vinaigrette, combine lemon juice, olive oil, salt, pepper, and stevia in a separate bowl.

Drizzle in dressing over-cooked carrots. Set aside.

Put together arugula, baby spinach, and roasted veggies in a salad bowl. Toss well to combine.

To serve, drizzle in just the right amount of vinaigrette over the salad.

Nutrition: Calories: 290; Fat: 9g; Fiber: 6g; Carbs: 6g; Protein: 32g.

50. Turmeric Tofu Scramble

Preparation Time: 10 minutes

Cooking Time: 15 minutes

Servings: 1

Ingredients:

- 1 portobello mushroom
- 3 or 4 cherry tomatoes
- ½ block tofu, firm
- ¼ tsp. ground turmeric
- 1 tsp. garlic powder
- Pepper and salt
- 1 tbsp. olive oil, some more for brushing

Directions:

Put the oven to a temperature of 400°F. Put the mushroom and tomatoes on a baking sheet and brush them with oil.
Sprinkle it with salt and pepper. Cook until tender, about 10 minutes.
In the meantime, mix tofu, turmeric, garlic powder, and a pinch of salt in a medium dish.
Mash with a fork.
In a large electric frying pan, over medium heat, put 1 tbsp. of olive oil. Add the tofu mixture and cook stirringly, until solid.

Nutrition: Calories: 451; Fat: 33g; Fiber: 2g; Carbs: 8g; Protein: 21g.

51. Raspberry Jam and Peanut Butter Overnight Oats

Preparation Time: 5 minutes

Cooking Time: 0 minutes

Servings: 2

Ingredients:

- ¼ cup easy-cooking rolled oats
- ½ cup 2-percent milk
- 1 tsp. sugar
- 3 tbsps. peanut butter, creamy
- 3 tbsps. raspberries, (whole)
- ¼ cup raspberries mashed

Directions:

In a medium bowl, combine oats, sugar, peanut butter, and squashed raspberries. Stir, until the batter is smooth.
Cover and chill overnight. In the morning, open and top with all the raspberries.

Nutrition: Calories: 234; Fat: 9g; Fiber: 2g; Carbs: 48g; Protein: 23g.

52. Roasted Broccoli with Lemon, Garlic and Toasted Pine Nuts

Preparation Time: 10 minutes

Cooking Time: 30 minutes

Servings: 2

Ingredients:

- 1 large head (1½ lbs.) broccoli, cut into stems and florets
- Freshly ground pepper
- Kosher salt
- 1 tsp. minced shallot
- ¼ cup olive oil (extra-virgin)
- 2 tsps. fresh lemon juice
- 1½ tbsps. pine nuts

Directions:

Settle the oven to 400°C. Place the broccoli flowers and stems on a wide baking sheet with 2 tablespoons. of olive oil and sprinkle with salt.

Bake the broccoli in the oven for around 30 minutes, stirring halfway through, till tender and browned.

Meanwhile, in a small pan, roast the pine nuts on moderate flame unless golden for approximately 4 minutes.

In a small pan, combine the lemon juice with a shallot and the leftover 2 tablespoons of olive oil; sprinkle with salt and pepper. Spread the broccoli in a serving dish. Then put the toasted nuts of pine and dressing, garnish well, and present.

Nutrition: Calories: 172; Fat: 8g; Fiber: 2g; Carbs: 8g; Protein: 6g.

53. Vegan Lentil Burger

Preparation Time: 10 minutes

Cooking Time: 45 minutes

Servings: 6

Ingredients:

- ¾ cup brown lentils
- 2 tsps. extra-virgin olive oil
- 1¾ cups low-sodium vegetable broth or water
- 1 large red onion, half thinly sliced and half chopped
- Lemon juice
- Kosher salt

- 8 oz. fresh spinach
- 2 large garlic cloves, minced
- Black pepper
- ½ tsp. ground cumin
- 1 cup whole-wheat bread crumbs
- Cooking spray
- ½ cup walnuts, toasted and finely chopped
- 6 whole-grain vegan buns

Directions:

Take the lentils and 1¾ cups of the broth for boiling at high temperature in a medium saucepan. Decrease heat to medium-low, partly covered, and cook until the lentils are entirely softened, and the liquid is absorbed for around 30 minutes.

Mix it with the leftover 1 tablespoon of the broth and mix well with the stick blender. Set it aside.

Warm the oil over medium temperature in a large non-stick skillet. Add the lemon juice, chopped onion, and ¼ teaspoon salt and cook for around 6 minutes, stirring till soft.

Add the spinach, garlic, 1 and a half teaspoon of black pepper and cumin, and stir until the spinach is withered for around 3 minutes.

Add the mixture of spinach, breadcrumbs, walnuts, and salt to the lentils and blend thoroughly. Put a cover and refrigerate for at least 1 hour or overnight.

Heat the grill to medium-high. Shape the mixture into 6 4-inch patties and sprinkle each side with a cooking spray. Grill till pleasant grill marks are formed, around 3 minutes per side. Put the patties in the buns with the chopped onion and other seasonings and eat.

Nutrition: Calories: 560; Fat: 14g; Fiber: 2g; Carbs: 65g; Protein: 21g.

54. Savory Oatmeal Bowl

Preparation Time: 10 minutes

Cooking Time: 10 minutes

Servings: 1

Ingredients:

- ½ cup old fashioned oatmeal
- 1 cup water
- 1 cooked egg
- 2 tbsps. grated parmesan cheese
- 3–4 grape tomatoes
- ¼ avocado
- Everything but The Bagel seasoning
- Sea salt and pepper
- Fresh herbs, for topping
- Hot sauce (optional)

Directions:

Heat the water and the oatmeal in a medium saucepan over lower temperatures.

Put a little sea salt in the oats. Prepare the oats, rolling periodically for 5-7 minutes or until the oats are smooth and the consistency you want.

In the meantime, cook your egg as much as you want, poached or fried is your preference.

When the oats and the eggs are cooked, take a bowl and put the oats and do the topping with cooked egg, avocado, parmesan cheese, everything but the bagel seasoning, fresh herbs, and hot sauce.

Nutrition: Calories: 330; Fat: 8g; Fiber: 16g; Carbs: 8g; Protein: 16g.

55. Vegan Coconut Kefir Banana Muffins

Preparation Time: 5 minutes

Cooking Time: 15 minutes

Servings: 6

Ingredients:

- 1½ cups all-purpose flour
- 1 cup crushed sugar
- 250 ml unsweetened shredded coconut
- 2 tsps. baking soda
- 1 tsp. baking powder

- ½ tsp. salt
- 2 ripe mashed bananas
- 1½ cups coconut milk, dairy-free
- 1 tsp. pure vanilla extract
- ¼ cup liquid coconut oil

Directions:

Settle the oven to 180°C. Sprinkle cooking spray on the muffin tin. Put it aside.

In a big bowl, whisk together sugar, flour, baking powder, shredded coconut, salt, and baking soda. Place it aside.

In a separate big cup, mix together bananas, vanilla, and coconut oil. Put the flour and mix, whisk until there are no white stripes left.

Add the mixture to the muffin pot. Keep baking till the upper parts are golden and the spatula put in the middle comes out clean, around 30 minutes. Allow chilling the muffin tin for 15 minutes.

Nutrition: Calories: 212; Fat: 7g; Fiber: 2g; Carbs: 35g; Protein: 2g.

56. Chicken Tetrazzini

Preparation Time: 15 minutes

Cooking Time: 25 minutes

Servings: 7

Ingredients:

- ¼ cup parmesan cheese, grated
- 1 cup mozzarella cheese, shredded
- 1 lb. chicken breast, boneless, skinless, & cubed

- 1 lb. whole wheat spaghetti noodles
- 1 medium onion, diced
- 1 tsp. oregano, dried

- 10 oz. button mushrooms, sliced
- 2 cups milk
- 2 medium bell peppers, diced
- 2 tbsps. extra virgin olive oil
- 3 cups chicken broth
- 3 large celery stalks, diced
- 3 tbsps. breadcrumbs
- Sea salt & pepper, to taste

Directions:

Warm a large pot or Dutch oven over medium heat and warm the oil in it.

Combine celery and onion into the pot, stirring completely to combine and allowing to cook for about 3 minutes or until shiny.

Stir the salt, pepper, mushrooms, peppers, and oregano into the pot and stir occasionally until all ingredients get shiny and begin to cook through.

Stir broth, milk, parmesan cheese, and chicken into the pot and stir until completely combined.

Break pasta noodles in half and stir them into the mixture, doing your best to get them spread evenly throughout the pot.

Cover and allow to cook for about 10 minutes.

In a medium mixing bowl, combine mozzarella and breadcrumbs, mixing completely.

Uncover the pot and stir once more before sprinkling the cheese and crumb mixture on top. Cover and let cook for about 3 to 5 more minutes, or until the cheese is nice and bubbly.

Serve hot!

Nutrition: Calories: 163; Fat: 8g; Fiber: 2g; Carbs: 8g; Protein: 11g.

57. Meatloaf

Preparation Time: 10 Minutes

Cooking Time: 40 Minutes

Servings: 9

Ingredients:

- 2 cups, ground beef
- 1 cup, ground chicken
- 2 eggs
- 1 tbsp. salt
- 1 tsp. ground black pepper
- ½ tsp. paprika
- 1 tbsp. butter
- 1 tsp. cilantro
- 1 tbsp. basil
- ¼ cup, fresh dill
- Breadcrumbs

Directions:

Combine chicken with ground beef in a mixing bowl.

Add egg, salt, ground black pepper, paprika, butter, cilantro, and basil.

Chop the dill and add it to the ground meat mixture and stir using your hand.

Place the meat mixture on aluminum foil and add breadcrumbs before wrapping it.

Place it in a pressure cooker and close its lid. Cook the dish in sauté mode and cook for 40 minutes.

When the cooking time ends, remove your meatloaf from the cooker and allow it to cool.

Unwrap the foil, slice it, and serve.

Nutrition: Calories: 173; Fat: 11.5g; Carbs: 0.81g; Protein: 16g.

58. Mixed Vegetables and Chicken Egg Rolls

Preparation Time: 10 minutes

Cooking Time: 15 minutes

Servings: 4

Ingredients:

- 1 tbsp. garlic, grated
- 1 tbsp. ginger, grated
- 4 tbsps. palm sugar, crumbled
- 1 banana chili, minced
- 4 tbsps. fish sauce
- 4 tbsps. rice wine vinegar
- 1 bird eye chili, minced
- 8 pieces spring roll wrappers
- Olive oil
- Water, for sealing
- 1 garlic clove, minced
- 1 shallot, julienned
- ¼ cup chicken, cooked shredded
- 1 cup bean sprouts
- 1 tbsp. chicken concentrate
- 2 tbsps. coconut oil
- ¼ cup squash, julienned
- ¼ cup carrots, julienned
- ¼ cup sweet potato, julienned
- ¼ cup potato, julienned
- ½ cup water
- A pinch of sea salt
- A pinch of black pepper

Directions:

Combine dipping sauce ingredients in a bowl. Stir until sugar dissolves. Taste; adjust seasoning if needed. Set aside.

To make spring rolls: pour coconut oil into a large wok set over medium heat. Sauté garlic and shallot until limp and transparent; except for bean sprouts, add in remaining filling ingredients. Cook until root crops are fork-tender. Toss in bean sprouts; stir. Turn off the heat immediately. Allow filling to cool completely to room temperature before rolling.

Add an equal portion of vegetable filling into spring roll paper; roll tightly, tucking in the edges and sealing with water. Set aside. Repeat step for remaining filling/wrapper.

Half-fill deep fryer with cooking oil set at medium heat. Cook only until spring rolls turn golden brown, about 7 minutes. Transfer cooked pieces on a plate lined with paper towels. Place 2 spring rolls on a plate; serve with dipping sauce on the side.

Nutrition: Calories: 260; Fat: 8g; Fiber: 1g; Carbs: 8g; Protein: 23g.

59. Chili Cod

Preparation Time: 10 minutes

Cooking Time: 12 minutes

Servings: 4

Ingredients:

- 4 cod fillets, boneless
- 2 tablespoons avocado oil

- A pinch of salt and black pepper
- 1 teaspoon chili powder
- 1 tablespoon cilantro, chopped
- 3 garlic cloves, minced
- ½ teaspoon chili pepper, crushed

Directions:
1. Heat up a pan with the oil over medium high heat, add the garlic, chili pepper and chili powder, stir and cook for 2 minutes.
2. Add the fish and the other ingredients, cook for 5 minutes on each side, divide between plates and serve.

Nutrition: calories 154, fat 3, fiber 0.5, carbs 4, protein 24

60. Parsley Tuna Bowls

Preparation Time: 10 minutes

Cooking Time: 14 minutes

Servings: 4

Ingredients:
- 1 pound tuna fillets, boneless, skinless and cubed
- 1 tablespoon olive oil
- 1 tablespoon parsley, chopped
- 2 scallions, chopped
- 1 tablespoon lime juice
- 1 teaspoon garlic powder
- A pinch of salt and black pepper

Directions:
1. Heat the oil in a pan over medium high heat, add the scallions and sauté for 2 minutes.
2. Add the fish and the other ingredients, toss gently, cook for 12 more minutes, divide into bowls and serve.

Nutrition: calories 447, fat 38.7, fiber 10.3, carbs 1.1, protein 24.1

CHAPTER 13: SOUPS

61. Creamy Broccoli and Cauliflower Soup

Preparation Time: 20 minutes

Cooking Time: 15 minutes

Servings: 6

Ingredients:

- 1 (13½ oz./383g) can unsweetened coconut milk
- 2 cups vegetable stock
- 1 (14 oz./397g) small head cauliflower, cored and cut into large florets
- 2 medium celery sticks, chopped
- 1 tsp. finely ground gray sea salt
- 6 green onions, green parts only, roughly chopped
- 1 large head broccoli, cored and cut into large florets
- ¼ tsp. ground black pepper
- ¼ tsp. ground white pepper
- ⅓ cup butter-infused olive oil
- 1 chopped green onion, for garnish

Directions:

Take a large saucepan and place it over medium heat.

Add coconut milk, vegetable stock, cauliflower florets, chopped celery, salt, and green onions.

Mix them gently, then cover and bring the soup to a boil.

Continue cooking the soup for 15 minutes until the cauliflower florets are soft.

Meanwhile, blanch the broccoli in a pot of boiling water for 1 minute until soft but still crisp, then drain on a paper towel. Set aside on a plate.

When the cauliflower soup is cooked, transfer it to a blender.

Add black pepper, white pepper, and olive oil. Blend the soup for 1 minute until smooth.

Add the soft broccoli and blend again for 30 seconds.

Divide the cooked broccoli and cauliflower soup into 6 serving bowls.

Garnish with chopped green onions and serve warm.

Nutrition: Calories: 264; Fat: 23.3g; Total Carbs: 10.3g; Fiber: 3.6g; Protein: 6.9g.

62. Chicken Turnip Soup

Preparation Time: 10 minutes

Cooking Time: 6 to 8 hours

Servings: 5

Ingredients:

- 12 oz. (340g) bone-in chicken
- ¼ cup turnip, chopped
- ¼ cup onions, chopped
- 4 garlic cloves, smashed
- 4 cups water
- 3 thyme sprigs
- 2 bay leaves
- Salt, to taste

- ¼ tsp. freshly ground black pepper

Directions:

Put the chicken, turnip, onions, garlic, water, thyme sprigs, and bay leaves in a slow cooker.
Season with salt and pepper, then give the mixture a good stir.
Cover and cook on low for 6 to 8 hours until the chicken is cooked through.
When ready, remove the bay leaves and shred the chicken with a fork.
Divide the soup among 5 bowls and serve.

Nutrition: Calories: 186; Fat: 13.6g; Total Carbs: 3.3g; Fiber: 2.6g; Protein: 15.2g

63. Garlicky Chicken Soup

Preparation Time: 10 minutes

Cooking Time: 10 minutes

Servings: 4

Ingredients:

- 2 tbsps. butter
- 1 large chicken breast cut into strips
- 4 oz. (113 g) cream cheese, cubed
- 2 tbsps. Garlic Gusto Seasoning
- ½ cup heavy cream
- 14½ oz. (411 g) chicken broth
- Salt, to taste

Directions:

Place a saucepan over medium heat and add butter to melt.
Add chicken strips and sauté for 2 minutes.
Add cream cheese and seasoning, and cook for 3 minutes, stirring occasionally.
Pour in the heavy cream and chicken broth. Bring the soup to a boil, then lower the heat.
Allow the soup to simmer for 4 minutes, then sprinkle with salt.
Let cool for 5 minutes and serve while warm.

Nutrition: Calories: 243; Fat: 22.5g; Total Carbs: 7.0g; Fiber: 6.6g; Protein: 9.6g.

64. Cauliflower Curry Soup

Preparation Time: 15 minutes

Cooking Time: 26 minutes

Servings: 4

Ingredients:

- 2 tbsps. avocado oil
- 1 white onion, chopped
- 4 garlic cloves, chopped
- ½ serrano pepper, seeds removed and chopped
- 1-inch ginger, chopped

- ¼ tsp. turmeric powder
- 2 tsps. curry powder
- ½ tsp. black pepper
- 1 tsp. salt
- 1 cup water
- 1 large cauliflower, cut into florets
- 1 cup chicken broth
- 1 can unsweetened coconut milk
- Cilantro, for garnish

Directions:

Place a saucepan over medium heat and add oil to heat.

Add onions to the hot oil and sauté them for 3 minutes.

Add garlic, Serrano pepper, and ginger, then sauté for 2 minutes.

Add turmeric, curry powder, black pepper, and salt. Cook for 1 minute after a gentle stir.

Pour water into the pan, then add cauliflower.

Cover this soup with a lid and cook for 10 minutes. Stir constantly.

Remove the soup from the heat and allow it to cool at room temperature.

Transfer this soup to a blender and purée the soup until smooth.

Return the soup to the saucepan and add broth and coconut milk. Cook for 10 minutes more and stir frequently.

Divide the soup into 4 bowls and sprinkle the cilantro on top for garnish before serving.

Nutrition: Calories: 342; Fat: 29.1g; Total Carbs: 18.3g; Fiber: 5.5g; Protein: 7.17g.

65. Beef Taco Soup

Preparation Time: 15 minutes

Cooking Time: 24 minutes

Servings: 8

Ingredients:

- 2 garlic cloves, minced
- ½ cup onions, chopped
- 1 lb. (454 g) ground beef
- 1 tsp. chili powder
- 1 tbsp. ground cumin
- 1 (8 oz./227g) package cream cheese, softened
- 2 (10 oz./284g) cans diced tomatoes and green chilies
- ½ cup heavy cream
- 2 tsps. salt
- 2 (14½ oz./411g) cans beef broth

Directions:

Take a large saucepan and place it over medium-high heat.

Add garlic, onions, and ground beef to the soup and sauté for 7 minutes until beef is browned.

Add chili powder and cumin, then cook for 2 minutes.

Add cream cheese and cook for 5 minutes while mashing the cream cheese into the beef with a spoon.

Add diced tomatoes and green chilies, heavy cream, salt and broth then cook for 10 minutes.

Mix gently and serve warm.

Nutrition: Calories: 205; Fat: 13.3g; Total Carbs: 4.4g; Fiber: 0.8g; Protein: 8.0g.

66. Creamy Tomato Soup

Preparation Time: 15 minutes

Cooking Time: 30 minutes

Servings: 4

Ingredients:

- 2 cups water
- 4 cups tomato juice
- 3 tomatoes, peeled, seeded and diced
- 14 leaves fresh basil
- 2 tbsps. butter
- 1 cup heavy whipping cream
- Salt and black pepper, to taste

Directions:

Take a suitable cooking pot and place it over medium heat.
Add water, tomato juice, and tomatoes, then simmer for 30 minutes.
Transfer the soup to a blender, then add basil leaves.
Press the pulse button and blend the soup until smooth.
Return this tomato soup to the cooking pot and place it over medium heat.
Add butter, heavy cream, salt, and black pepper. Cook and mix until the butter melts.
Serve warm and fresh.

Nutrition: Calories: 203; Fat: 17.7g; Total Carbs: 13.0g; Fiber: 5.6g; Protein: 3.7g.

67. Creamy Broccoli and Leek Soup

Preparation Time: 5 minutes

Cooking Time: 25 minutes

Servings: 4

Ingredients:

- 10 oz. broccoli
- 1 leek
- 8 oz. cream cheese
- 3 oz. butter
- 3 cups water
- 1 garlic clove
- ½ cup fresh basil
- Salt and pepper

Directions:

Rinse the leek and chop both parts finely. Slice the broccoli thinly.
Place the veggies in a pot and cover with water and then season them. Boil the water until the broccoli softens.
Add the florets and garlic, while lowering the heat.
Add in the cheese, butter, pepper, and basil. Blend until desired consistency: if too thick use water; if you want to make it thicker, use a little bit of heavy cream.

Nutrition: Calories: 451; Fats: 37g; Protein: 10g; Carbs: 4g.

68. Chicken Soup

Preparation Time: 25 minutes

Cooking Time: 1 hour and 25 minutes

Servings: 4

Ingredients:

- 6 cups water
- 1 chicken
- 1 medium carrot
- 1 yellow onion
- 1 bay leaf
- 1 leek

- 2 garlic cloves
- 1 tbsp. dried thyme
- ½ cup white wine, dry (no, not for drinking)
- 1 tsp. peppercorns
- Salt and pepper

Directions:

Peel and cut your veggies. Brown them in oil in a big pot.

Split your chicken in half, down in the middle. Pour water and spices into the pot. Let it simmer for 1 hour.

Take out the chicken save the meat, and toss away the bones.

Put the meat back in the pot, and let it simmer on medium heat for 20-25 minutes again, while seasoning to your liking.

Nutrition: Calories: 145; Fats: 12g; Carbs: 1g; Protein: 8g.

69. Wild Mushroom Soup

Preparation Time: 10 minutes

Cooking Time: 30 minutes

Servings: 4

Ingredients:

- 6 oz. mix portabella mushrooms, oyster mushrooms, and shiitake mushrooms
- 3 cups water
- 1 garlic clove
- 1 shallot

- 4 oz. butter
- 1 chicken bouillon cube
- ½ lb. celery root
- 1 tbsp. white wine vinegar
- 1 cup heavy whipping cream
- Fresh parsley

Directions:

Clean, trim, and chop your mushrooms and celery. Do the same to your shallot and garlic.

Sauté your chopped veggies in butter over medium heat in a saucepan.

Add thyme, vinegar, chicken bouillon cube, and water as you bring to a boil. Then let it simmer for 10-15 minutes.

Add cream to them with an immersion blender until your desired consistency. Serve with parsley on top.

Nutrition: Calories: 481; Fats: 47g; Protein: 7g; Carbs: 9g.

70. Roasted Butternut Squash Soup

Preparation Time: 15 minutes

Cooking Time: 43 minutes

Servings: 4

Ingredients:

- 1 large butternut squash, cubed and peeled
- 1 stalk celery, sliced
- 2 potatoes, peeled, chopped
- 1 onion, chopped
- 1 large carrot, chopped
- 3 tbsps. olive oil
- 1 tbsp. fresh thyme
- 25 oz. chicken broth
- 1 tbsp. butter
- Salt and pepper

Directions:

Preheat your oven to 400°F. On a baking sheet, toss squash and potatoes with 2 tbsps. oil and season to your taster. Roast for 20-25 minutes.

In the meantime, melt your butter and the rest of the oil in a large pot over medium heat. Add the onion, celery, carrot, and cook for 5-8 minutes. Season them, too.

Add roasted squash and potatoes. Then pour over the chicken broth. Simmer it for 10 minutes using an immersion blender until the soup is creamy.

Garnish it with thyme.

Nutrition: Calories: 254; Fats: 15g; Carbs: 19g; Protein: 6g.

71. Zucchini Cream Soup

Preparation Time: 5 minutes

Cooking Time: 20 minutes

Servings: 4

Ingredients:

- 3 zucchinis
- 32 oz. chicken broth
- 2 cloves garlic
- 2 tbsps. sour cream
- ½ small onion
- Parmesan cheese (for topping if desired)

Directions:

Combine your broth, garlic, zucchini, and onion in a large pot over medium heat until boiling.

Lower the heat, cover, and let simmer for 15-20 minutes

Remove from heat and purée with an immersion blender, while adding the sour cream and pureeing until smooth.

Season to taste and top with your cheese.

Nutrition: Calories: 117; Fats: 9g; Carbs: 3g; Protein: 4g.

72. Cauli Soup

Preparation Time: 5 minutes

Cooking Time: 25 minutes

Servings: 6

Ingredients:

- 32 oz. vegetable broth
- 1 head cauli, diced
- 2 garlic cloves, minced
- 1 onion, diced
- ½ tbsp. olive oil
- Salt and pepper
- Grated parmesan, sliced green onion for topping

Directions:

In a pot, heat oil over medium heat, while adding the onion and garlic. Then cook them for 4-5 minutes.
Add in the cauli and vegetable broth. Boil it and then cover for 15-20 minutes while covered.
Pour all contents of the pot into a blender and season it.
Blend until smooth. Top it with your cheese and green onion.

Nutrition: Calories: 37; Fats: 1g; Carbs: 3g; Protein: 3g.

73. Thai Coconut Soup

Preparation Time: 10 minutes

Cooking Time: 35 minutes

Servings: 4

Ingredients:

- 3 chicken breasts
- 9 oz. coconut milk
- 9 oz. chicken broth
- ⅔ tbsps. chili sauce
- 18 oz. water
- ⅔ tbsps. coconut aminos
- ⅔ oz. lime juice
- ⅔ tsps. ground ginger
- ¼ cup red boat fish sauce
- Salt and pepper

Directions:

Slice up the chicken breasts thinly. Make them bite-sized.
In a large stockpot, mix your coconut milk, water, fish sauce, chili sauce, lime juice, ginger, coconut aminos, and broth. Bring to a boil.
Stir in chicken pieces. Then reduce the heat and cover the pot, while simmering it for 30 minutes.
Remove the basil leaves and season them.

Nutrition: Calories: 227; Fats: 17g; Carbs: 3g; Protein: 19g.

74. Chicken Ramen Soup

Preparation Time: 10 minutes

Cooking Time: 20 minutes

Servings: 2

Ingredients:

- 1 chicken breast
- 2 eggs
- 1 zucchini, made into noodles
- 4 cups chicken broth
- 2 cloves garlic, peeled and minced
- 2 tbsps. coconut aminos
- 3 tbsps. avocado oil
- 1 tbsp. ginger

Directions:

Pan-fry the chicken in avocado oil in a pan until brown.

Hard boil your eggs and slice them in half.

Add chicken broth to a large pot and simmer with the garlic, coconut aminos, and ginger. Then add in the zucchini noodles for 4-5 minutes.

Put the broth into a bowl, top it with eggs and chicken slices, and season to your liking.

Nutrition: Calories: 478; Fats: 39g; Carbs: 3g; Protein: 31g.

CHAPTER 14: DESSERTS

75. Baked Apples

Preparation Time: 15 minutes | **Cooking Time:** 18 minutes | **Servings:** 4

Ingredients:

- 4 apples, cored
- ¼ cup coconut oil, softened
- 4 tsps. ground cinnamon
- ⅛ tsp. ground ginger
- ⅛ tsp. ground nutmeg

Directions:

Preheat the oven to 350°F.
Fill each apple with 1 tbsp. of coconut oil.
Sprinkle with spices evenly.
Arrange the apples on a baking sheet.
Bake for about 12-18 minutes.

Nutrition: Calories: 240; Total Fat: 14.1g; Saturated Fat: 11.8g; Cholesterol: 0mg; Sodium: 2mg; Total Carbs: 32.7g; Fiber: 6.6g; Sugar: 23.3g; Protein: 0.7g.

76. Pumpkin Ice Cream

Preparation Time: 15 minutes | **Cooking Time:** 0 minutes | **Servings:** 6

Ingredients:

- 15 oz. homemade pumpkin puree
- ½ cup dates, pitted and chopped
- 2 (14-oz) cans unsweetened coconut milk
- ½ tsp. organic vanilla extract
- 1½ tsp. pumpkin pie spice
- ½ tsp. ground cinnamon
- A pinch of sea salt

Directions:

In a high-speed blender, add all the ingredients and pulse until smooth.
Transfer into an airtight container and freeze for about 1-2 hours.
Now, transfer the mixture into an ice cream maker and process it according to the manufacturer's directions.
Return the ice cream to the airtight container and freeze for about 1-2 hours before serving.

Nutrition: Calories: 293; Total Fat: 22.5g; Saturated Fat: 20.1g; Cholesterol: 0mg; Sodium: 99mg; Total Carbs: 24.8g; Fiber: 3.6g; Sugar: 14.1g; Protein: 2.3g.

77. Avocado Pudding

Preparation Time: 15 minutes   **Cooking Time:** 0 minutes   **Servings:** 4

Ingredients:

- 2 cups bananas, peeled and chopped
- 2 ripe avocados, peeled, pitted, and chopped
- 1 tsp. fresh lime zest, grated finely
- 1 tsp. fresh lemon zest, grated finely
- ½ cup fresh lime juice
- ½ cup fresh lemon juice
- ⅓ cup agave nectar

Directions:

In a blender, add all the ingredients and pulse until smooth.
Transfer the mousse into 4 serving glasses and refrigerate to chill for about 3 hours before serving.

Nutrition: Calories: 462; Total Fat: 20.1g; Saturated Fat: 4.4g; Cholesterol: 0mg; Sodium: 13mg; Total Carbs: 48.2g; Fiber: 10.2g; Sugar 30.4g; Protein: 3g.

78. Chocolate Mousse

Preparation Time: 10 minutes   **Cooking Time:** 0 minutes   **Servings:** 4

Ingredients:

- ½ cup unsweetened almond milk
- 1 cup cooked black beans
- 4 Medjool dates, pitted and chopped
- ½ cup pecans, chopped
- 2 tbsps. non-alkalized cocoa powder
- 1 tsp. organic vanilla extract
- 4 tbsps. fresh blueberries

Directions:

In a food processor, add all the ingredients and pulse until smooth and creamy.
Transfer the mixture into serving bowls and refrigerate to chill before serving.
Garnish with blueberries and serve.

Nutrition: Calories: 357; Total Fat: 13g; Saturated Fat: 1.7g; Cholesterol: 0mg; Sodium: 26mg; Total Carbs: 52.1g; Fiber: 11.9g; Sugar: 16.7g; Protein: 13.4g.

79. Apple Crisp

Preparation Time: 15 minutes   **Cooking Time:** 20

minutes   **Servings:** 8

Ingredients:

For Filling:

- 2 large apples, peeled, cored, and chopped
- 2 tbsps. water
- 2 tbsps. fresh apple juice
- ¼ tsp. ground cinnamon

For Topping:

- ½ cup quick rolled oats
- ¼ cup unsweetened coconut flakes
- 2 tbsps. pecans, chopped
- ½ tsp. ground cinnamon
- ¼ cup water

Directions:

Preheat the oven to 300°F. Lightly grease a baking dish.
To make the filling add all of the ingredients to a large bowl and gently mix. Set this aside.
Make the topping by adding all of the ingredients to another bowl and mix well.
Place the filling mixture into the prepared baking dish then spread the topping over the filling mixture evenly.
Bake for about 20 minutes or until the top becomes golden brown.
Serve warm.

Nutrition: Calories: 100; Total Fat: 2.7g; Saturated Fat: 0.8g; Cholesterol: 0mg; Sodium: 3mg; Total Carbs: 19.1g; Fiber: 2.6g; Sugar: 11.9g; Protein: 1.2g.

80. Chocolate Crunch Bars

Preparation Time: 5 minutes   **Cooking Time:** 3 minutes   **Servings:** 4

Ingredients:

- 1½ cups sugar-free chocolate chips
- 1 cup almond butter
- Stevia to taste
- ¼ cup coconut oil
- 3 cups pecans, chopped

Directions:

Layer an 8-inch baking pan with parchment paper.
Mix chocolate chips with butter, coconut oil, and sweetener in a bowl.
Melt it by heating in a microwave for 2 to 3 minutes until well mixed.
Stir in nuts and seeds. Mix gently.
Pour this batter into the baking pan and spread evenly.
Refrigerate for 2 to 3 hours.
Slice and serve.

Nutrition: Calories: 316; Total Fat: 30.9g; Saturated Fat: 8.1g; Cholesterol: 0mg; Total Carbs: 8.3g; Sugar: 1.8g; Fiber: 3.8g; Sodium: 8mg; Protein: 6.4g.

81. Homemade Protein Bar

Preparation Time: 5 minutes   **Cooking Time:** 0 minutes   **Servings:** 4

Ingredients:

- 1 cup nut butter
- 4 tbsps. coconut oil
- 2 scoops vanilla protein
- Stevia, to taste
- ½ tsp. sea salt
- 1 tsp. cinnamon (Optional)

Directions:

Mix coconut oil with butter, protein, stevia, and salt in a dish.
Stir in cinnamon and chocolate chip.
Press the mixture firmly and freeze until firm.
Cut the crust into small bars.
Serve and enjoy.

Nutrition: Calories: 179; Total Fat: 15.7g; Saturated Fat: 8g; Cholesterol: 0mg; Total Carbs: 4.8g; Sugar: 3.6g; Fiber: 0.8g; Sodium: 43mg; Protein: 5.6g.

82. Shortbread Cookies

Preparation Time: 10 minutes   **Cooking Time:** 15 minutes   **Servings:** 6

Ingredients:

- 2½ cups almond flour
- 6 tbsps. nut butter
- ½ cup erythritol
- 1 tsp. vanilla essence

Directions:

Preheat your oven to 350°F.
Layer a cookie sheet with parchment paper.
Beat butter with erythritol until fluffy.
Stir in vanilla essence and almond flour. Mix well until becomes crumbly.
Spoon out a tablespoon of cookie dough onto the cookie sheet.
Add more dough to make as many cookies.
Bake for 15 minutes until brown.
Serve.

Nutrition: Calories: 288; Total Fat: 25.3g; Saturated Fat: 6.7g; Cholesterol: 23mg; Total Carbs: 9.6g; Sugar: 0.1g; Fiber: 3.8g; Sodium: 74mg; Potassium: 3mg; Protein: 7.6g.

83. Peanut Butter Bars

Preparation Time: 10 minutes **Cooking Time:** 0 minutes **Servings:** 6

Ingredients:

- ¾ cup almond flour
- 2 oz. almond butter
- ¼ cup Swerve
- ½ cup peanut butter
- ½ tsp. vanilla

Directions:

Combine all the ingredients for bars.
Transfer this mixture to a 6-inch small pan. Press it firmly.
Refrigerate for 30 minutes.
Slice and serve.

Nutrition: Calories: 214; Total Fat: 19g; Saturated Fat: 5.8g; Cholesterol: 15mg; Total Carbs: 6.5g; Sugar: 1.9g; Fiber: 2.1g; Sodium: 123mg; Protein: 6.5g.

84. Zucchini Bread Pancakes

Preparation Time: 15 minutes **Cooking Time:** 8 minutes **Servings:** 3

Ingredients:

- 1 tbsp. grapeseed oil
- ½ cup chopped walnuts
- 2 cups walnut milk
- 1 cup shredded zucchini
- ¼ cup mashed burro banana
- 2 tbsps. date sugar
- 2 cup kamut flour or spelled

Directions:

Place the date sugar and flour into a bowl. Whisk together.
Add in the mashed banana and walnut milk. Stir until combined. Remember to scrape the bowl to get all the dry mixture. Add in walnuts and zucchini. Stir well until combined.
Place the grapeseed oil onto a griddle and warm.
Pour ¼ cup batter on the hot griddle. Leave it along until bubbles begin forming on to surface. Carefully turn over the pancake and cook for another 4 minutes until cooked through.
Place the pancakes onto a serving plate and enjoy with some agave syrup.

Nutrition: Calories: 246; Carbs: 49.2g; Fiber: 4.6g; Protein: 7.8g.

85. Berry Sorbet

Preparation Time: 10 minutes **Cooking Time:** 10 minutes **Servings:** 6

Ingredients:

- 2 cups water
- 2 cups blend strawberries
- 1½ tsp. spelled flour
- ½ cup date sugar

Directions:

Pour the water into a large pot and let the water begin to warm. Add the flour and date sugar and stir until dissolved. Allow this mixture to start boiling and continue to cook for around 10 minutes. It should have started to thicken. Take off heat and set to the side to cool.
Once the syrup has cooled off, add in the strawberries, and stir well to combine.
Pour into a container that is freezer safe and put it into the freezer until frozen.
Take sorbet out of the freezer, cut into chunks, and put it either into a blender or a food processor. Hit the pulse button until the mixture is creamy.
Pour this into the same freezer-safe container and put it back into the freezer for 4 hours.

Nutrition: Calories: 99; Carbs: 8g; Fiber: 6.7g; Protein: 12.8g

86. Quinoa Porridge

Preparation Time: 5 minutes **Cooking Time:** 15 minutes **Servings:** 4

Ingredients:

- Zest 1 lime
- ½ cup coconut milk
- ½ tsp. cloves
- 1½ tsp. ground ginger
- 2 cup spring water
- 1 cup quinoa
- 1 grated apple

Directions:

Cook the quinoa according to the instructions on the package. When the quinoa has been cooked, drain well. Put it back into the pot and stir in spices.
Add coconut milk and stir well to combine.
Grate the apple now and stir well.
Divide equally into bowls and add the lime zest on top. Sprinkle with nuts and seeds of choice.

Nutrition: Calories: 180; Fat: 3g; Carbs: 40g; Protein: 10g.

87. Apple Quinoa

Preparation Time: 15 minutes

Cooking Time: 15 minutes

Servings: 4

Ingredients:

- 1 tbsp. coconut oil
- Ginger
- ½ key lime

- 1 apple
- ½ cup quinoa

Optional Toppings:

- Seeds
- Nuts
- Berries

Directions:

Fix the quinoa according to the instructions on the package. When you are getting close to the end of the cooking time, grate in the apple and cook for 30 seconds.
Zest the lime into the quinoa and squeeze the juice in. Stir in the coconut oil.
Divide evenly into bowls and sprinkle with some ginger.
You can add in some berries, nuts, and seeds right before you eat.

Nutrition: Calories: 146; Fiber: 2.3g; Fat: 8.3g; Carbs: 15.6g; Protein: 1.5g.

88. Kamut Porridge

Preparation Time: 10 minutes

Cooking Time: 25 minutes

Servings: 4

Ingredients:

- 4 tbsps. agave syrup
- 1 tbsp. coconut oil
- ½ tsp. sea salt

- 1 cup coconut milk
- 1 cup kamut berries

Optional Toppings:

- Berries
- Coconut chips

- Ground nutmeg
- Ground cloves

Directions:

You need to "crack" the Kamut berries. You can do this by placing the berries into a food processor and pulsing until you have 1¼ cups of Kamut.

Put the cracked Kamut in a pot with salt and coconut milk. Give it a good stir to combine everything. Allow this mixture to come to a full rolling boil and then turn the heat down until the mixture is simmering. Stir every now and then until the Kamut has thickened to your likeness. This normally takes about 10 minutes.

Take off heat, stir in agave syrup and coconut oil.

Garnish with toppings of choice and enjoy.

Nutrition: Calories: 114; Protein: 5g; Carbs: 24g; Fiber: 4g.

---

89. Overnight "Oats"

Preparation Time: 5 minutes

Cooking Time: 0 minutes

Servings: 4

Ingredients:

- ½ cup berries
- ½ burro banana
- ½ tsp. ginger
- ½ cup coconut milk
- ½ cup hemp seeds

Directions:

Put the hemp seeds, salt, and coconut milk into a glass jar. Mix well.

Place the lid on the jar and put it in the refrigerator to sit overnight.

The next morning, add the ginger, berries, and banana. Stir well and enjoy.

Nutrition: Calories: 139; Fat: 4.1g; Protein: 9g; Sugar: 7g.

---

90. Blueberry Cupcakes

Preparation Time: 15 minutes

Cooking Time: 30 minutes

Servings: 4

Ingredients:

- Grapeseed oil
- ½ tsp. sea salt
- ¼ cup sea moss gel
- ⅓ cup agave
- ½ cup blueberries
- ¾ cup teff flour
- ¾ cup spelled flour
- 1 cup coconut milk

Directions:

Heat your oven to 365°. Place paper liners into a muffin tin.

Place sea moss gel, sea salt, agave, flour, and milk in a large bowl. Mix well to combine. Gently fold in blueberries.

Gently pour batter into paper liners. Place in oven and bake for 30 minutes.

They are done when they have turned a nice golden color, and they spring back when you touch them.

Nutrition: Calories: 85; Fat: 0.7g; Carbs: 12g; Protein: 1.4g; Fiber: 5g.

91. Brazil Nut Cheese

Preparation Time: 2 hours

Cooking Time: 0 minutes

Servings: 4

Ingredients:

- 2 tsps. grapeseed oil
- 1½ cups water
- 1½ cups hemp milk
- ½ tsp. cayenne
- 1 tsp. onion powder

- Juice ½ lime
- 2 tsps. sea salt
- 1 lb. Brazil nuts
- 1 tsp. onion powder

Directions:

You will need to start by soaking the Brazil nuts in some water. You just put the nuts into a bowl and make sure the water covers them. Soak no less than 2 hours or overnight. Overnight would be best.

Now you need to put everything except water into a food processor or blender.

Add just ½ cups water and blend for 2 minutes

Continue adding ½ cup water and blending until you have the consistency you want.

Scrape into an airtight container and enjoy.

Nutrition: Calories: 187; Protein: 4.1g; Fat: 19g; Carbs: 3.3g; Fiber: 2.1g.

CHAPTER 15: SNACKS

---

92. Squash Bites

Preparation Time: 10 minutes | **Cooking Time:** 40 minutes | **Servings:** 4

Ingredients:

- 10 oz. turkey meat, cooked, sliced
- 2 lbs. butternut squash, cubed
- 1 tsp. chili powder
- 1 tsp. garlic powder
- 1 tsp. sweet paprika
- Black pepper to taste

Directions:

In a bowl, mix butternut squash cubes with chili powder, black pepper, garlic powder, and paprika, and toss to coat.

Wrap squash pieces in turkey slices, place them all on a lined baking sheet, place in the oven at 350°F, bake for 20 minutes, flip and bake for 20 minutes more.

Arrange squash bites on a platter and serve.

Enjoy!

Nutrition: Calories: 223; Fat: 3.8g; Fiber: 4.5g; Carbs: 26.5g; Protein: 23g.

---

93. Pepperoni Bites

Preparation Time: 5 minutes | **Cooking Time:** 10 minutes | **Servings:** 24 pieces

Ingredients:

- ⅓ cup tomatoes, chopped
- ½ cup bell peppers, mixed and chopped
- 24 pepperoni slices
- ½ cup tomato sauce
- 4 oz. almond cheese, cubed
- 2 tbsps. basil, chopped
- Black pepper to taste

Directions:

Divide pepperoni slices into a muffin tray.

Divide tomato and bell pepper pieces into the pepperoni cups.

Also divide the tomato sauce, basil, and almond cheese cubes, sprinkle black pepper at the end, place cups in the oven at 400°F, and bake for 10 minutes.

Arrange the pepperoni bites on a platter and serve.

Enjoy!

Nutrition: Calories: 59; Fat: 4.5g; Fiber: 0.1g; Carbs: 2g; Protein: 2.5g.

94. Party Meatballs

Preparation Time: 10 minutes   **Cooking Time:** 8 minutes   **Servings:** 20

Ingredients:

- 1 lb. turkey meat, ground
- 1 tbsp. coconut oil, melted
- 1 yellow onion, chopped
- 1 egg
- 1 cup coconut flour
- 1 tsp. Italian seasoning
- A pinch sea salt
- Black pepper to taste
- 2 tbsps. parsley, chopped

Directions:

In a bowl, mix turkey meat with half of the flour, a pinch of salt, black pepper, Italian seasoning, parsley, onion, egg, and hot sauce and stir well.

Put the rest of the flour in another bowl.

Shape 20 turkey meatballs and dip each 1 in flour.

Heat up a pan with the oil over medium-high heat, add meatballs, cook them for 4 minutes on each side, transfer to paper towels to remove any excess grease, place all of them on a platter and serve.

Enjoy!

Nutrition: Calories: 71; Fat: 2.6g; Fiber: 2.2g; Carbs: 4.1g; Protein: 7.7g.

95. Artichoke Petals Bites

Preparation Time: 10 minutes   **Cooking Time:** 10 minutes   **Servings:** 8

Ingredients:

- 8 oz. artichoke petals, boiled, drained, without salt
- ½ cup almond flour
- 4 oz. parmesan, grated
- 2 tbsps. almond butter, melted

Directions:

In the mixing bowl, mix up together almond flour and grated Parmesan.

Preheat the oven to 355°F.

Dip the artichoke petals in the almond butter and then coat in the almond flour mixture.

Place them in the tray.

Transfer the tray to the preheated oven and cook the petals for 10 minutes.

Chill the cooked petal bites a little before serving.

Nutrition: Calories: 93; Protein: 6.54g; Fat: 3.72g; Carbs: 9.08g.

96. Stuffed Beef Loin in Sticky Sauce

Preparation Time: 15 minutes

Cooking Time: 40 minutes

Servings: 4

Ingredients:

- 1 tbsp. erythritol
- 1 tbsp. lemon juice
- 1 tbsp. butter
- ½ tsp. tomato sauce
- ¼ tsp. dried rosemary
- 9 oz. beef loin
- 3 oz. celery root, grated

- 3 oz. bacon, sliced
- 1 tbsp. walnuts, chopped
- ¾ tsp. garlic, diced
- 2 tsps. butter
- 1 tbsp. olive oil
- 1 tsp. salt
- ½ cup water

Directions:

Cut the beef loin into the layer and spread it with the dried rosemary, butter, and salt. Then place over the beef loin: grated celery root, sliced bacon, walnuts, and diced garlic.

Roll the beef loin and brush it with olive oil. Secure the meat with the help of the toothpicks. Place it in the tray and add a ½ cup of water.

Cook the meat in the preheated to 365°F oven for 40 minutes.

Meanwhile, make the sticky sauce: Mix up together Erythritol, lemon juice, 4 tablespoons of water, and butter. Preheat the mixture until it starts to boil. Then add tomato sauce and whisk it well.

Bring the sauce to boil and remove from the heat.

When the beef loin is cooked, remove it from the oven and brush it with the cooked sticky sauce very generously.

Slice the beef roll and sprinkle with the remaining sauce.

Nutrition: Calories: 321; Protein: 18.35g; Fat: 26.68g; Carbs: 2.75g.

97. Eggplant Fries

Preparation Time: 10 minutes

Cooking Time: 15 minutes

Servings: 8

Ingredients:

- 2 eggs
- 2 cups almond flour
- 2 tbsps. coconut oil, spray

- 2 eggplant, peeled and cut thinly
- Salt and pepper

Directions:

Preheat your oven to 400°F.

Take a bowl and mix with salt and black pepper in it

Take another bowl and beat eggs until frothy

Dip the eggplant pieces into eggs
Then coat them with a flour mixture
Add another layer of flour and egg
Then, take a baking sheet and grease it with coconut oil on top
Bake for about 15 minutes
Serve and enjoy.

Nutrition: Calories: 212; Fat: 15.8g; Carbs: 12.1g; Protein: 8.6g

98. Parmesan Crisps

Preparation Time: 5 minutes

Cooking Time: 5 minutes

Servings: 8

Ingredients:

- 1 tsp. butter

- 8 oz. parmesan cheese, full fat and shredded

Directions:

Preheat your oven to 400°F
Put parchment paper on a baking sheet and grease with butter
Spoon parmesan into 8 mounds, spreading them apart evenly
Flatten them
Bake for 5 minutes until browned
Let them cool
Serve and enjoy.

Nutrition: Calories: 133; Fat: 11g; Carbs: 1g; Protein: 11g

99. Roasted Broccoli

Preparation Time: 5 minutes

Cooking Time: 20 minutes

Servings: 4

Ingredients:

- 4 cups broccoli florets
- 1 tbsp. olive oil

- Salt and pepper to taste

Directions:

Preheat your oven to 400°F
Add broccoli in a zip bag alongside oil and shake until coated

Add seasoning and shake again
Spread broccoli out on the baking sheet, bake for 20 minutes
Let it cool and serve.

Nutrition: Calories: 62, Fat: 4g; Carbs: 4g; Protein: 4g.

100. Almond Flour Muffins

Preparation Time: 15 minutes

Cooking Time: 30 minutes

Servings: 8

Ingredients:

- ⅓ cup pumpkin puree
- 3 eggs
- 2 tbsps. agave nectar
- 2 tbsps. coconut oil
- 1 tsp. vanilla extract
- 1 tsp. white vinegar
- 1 cup chopped fruits
- 1 tsp. baking soda
- ½ tsp. salt

Directions:

Preheat the oven to 350°F.
Line the muffin tin with paper liners
In the first mixing bowl, whisk the almond flour, salt, and baking soda.
In the second mixing bowl, whisk the pumpkin puree, eggs, coconut oil, agave nectar, vanilla extract, and vinegar.
Now add this puree mix of the second bowl to the first bowl and blend everything well.
Add the chopped fruits to the blend.
Pour the mixture into the muffin cups in your pan.
Bake for 15-20 minutes. Ensure that the contents have been set in the center, and a golden-brown lining has started to appear at the edges.
Transfer the muffins to a cooling rack and let them cool completely.

Nutrition: Calories: 75; Carbs: 4g; Fat: 6g; Protein: 0g.

Conclusion

Many people have found benefits from fasting, no matter their age. Women, in particular, may feel that they will not lose weight or be able to stick with the diet. They might even hear the criticism of other women who are doing it: "You're too old to be doing this!"

In reality, intermittent fasting can help you lose weight, have more energy, and gain a better connection with your body. Women over the age of 50 find it easier to fast than men of the same age because they have a lower risk of health complications and do not lose as much muscle mass while fasting as men do. There are two different forms of intermittent fasting known as the 16:8 method and the 5:2 method.

In the 16:8 method, you fast for 16 hours and then only eat for 8 hours. You can break up the fasting period any way that works best for your schedule. For example, you could choose to stop eating at 8 pm and start eating again at 12 pm. This will require a lot of discipline at first because it is hard to go that long without food!

If you're just getting started with intermittent fasting, this is a great place to start. To stay within your recommended daily intake, you should keep track of your calories even when you aren't eating.

In the 5:2 method, you fast for two days a week. For example, you would eat whatever you wanted on Monday and then eat very little on Tuesday and Wednesday.

The key is to eat as little as possible on non-fasting days so that your body can burn fat while you sleep without having to worry about digestion. You should drink lots of water before bed to help with sleep and dehydration. Five days out of the week, it is recommended that you consume carbohydrates after exercising or at night before going to bed to replenish muscle glycogen.

Another benefit of this method is that it can help women with irregular cycles have more regular periods. However, if you are going to try this method, slowly transition to it starting on the day of the fast. By taking the first 24 hours off from eating in order to begin with, you will be able to better regulate your period so that it doesn't become irregular.

A lot of people say that this should only be done once or twice a year, but for some women, it can work year-round because the effect is cumulative on your metabolism. After about three months of fasting, many women will start losing at least 10 pounds.

When you cut calories, your body will start to consume adipose tissue. You should be prepared for a reduction in energy levels because this is the time when women will start to feel hungry. Just remember that you aren't doing this so that you can eat a lot; you are doing it so that you can be healthy and lose weight.

As soon as enough adipose tissue has been burned off, you will notice an improvement in your energy levels and endurance. During the fast, try to move around for at least 20 minutes a day, but do not exercise because that will break the fast too quickly. Yoga is usually the best exercise for women who are just starting out with fasting since it doesn't involve doing anything too vigorous.

Your body will start to adapt to eating less beginning on day eight of fasting. Once your body has adjusted, you should be able to maintain your weight loss and have healthy periods.

Manufactured by Amazon.ca
Bolton, ON

29223362R00057